ANIMAL DISEASE SURVEILLANCE AND SURVEY SYSTEMS

Methods and Applications

Animal Disease Surveillance and Survey Systems

Methods and Applications

Edited by

M. D. Salman

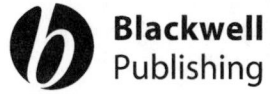
Blackwell Publishing

M. D. SALMAN is Professor of Veterinary Epidemiology at Colorado State University's Animal Population Health Institute, College c~~f Veterinary Medicine and Biomedical Science~~

© 2003 Iowa State Press
A Blackwell Publishing Compa~~ny~~

Blackwell Publishing Professional
2121 State Avenue, Ames, Iowa 50014

Orders: 1-800-862-6657
Office: 1-515-292-0140
Fax: 1-515-292-3348
Web site: www.blackwellprofessiona~~l.com~~

Printed on acid-free paper in the United States of America

First edition, 2003

Library of Congress Cataloging-in-Publication Data

Salman, Mowafak Dauod.
    Animal disease surveillance and survey systems: methods and applications/by M.D.
      Salman.—1st ed.
        p. ; cm.
Includes bibliographical references and index.
    ISBN 0-8138-1031-0 (alk. paper)
  1. Veterinary epidemiology.
    [DNLM: 1. Animal Diseases—epidemiology.   2. Sentinel
Surveillance—veterinary. SF 780.9 S171a 2003]   I. Title.
    SF780.9.S25 2003
    636.089'4—dc21

2003013531

The last digit is the print number: 9 8 7 6 5 4 3 2

Table of Contents

Preface

Most of the textbooks for epidemiology and veterinary medicine mentioned surveillance and survey as approaches to monitor and subsequently prevent the spread of diseases. Most of these books, however, assume that readers and users of epidemiology have the knowledge to excuse scientifically based plan for surveillance program. There are several methodological issues that need to be considered before such planning. Although some of these issues have been addressed in some of these textbooks, their relevant values to surveillance or monitoring were not included. Furthermore, most of these excellent books in epidemiology and preventive medicine have ignored the potential implementers and users of surveillance programs—specifically, government, international organizations, and public health agencies. Such users may require different ways to present information with more instruction on how to do it and fewer academic concepts. This book attempts to satisfy the requirements for an effective and scientifically sound surveillance for animal diseases or other health issues. Both concepts and examples are given for several of the approaches to such surveillance systems. The intention is to avoid in-depth academic elaboration of specific issues, as such elaboration is found in other classical textbooks.

Mo Salman

Acknowledgments

This book has been influenced by many people. I wish to gratefully acknowledge the dedication of the contributors to this book. They are the essential nucleus for this book—without their input, this book would not have been published. My special thanks to Ian Gardner, who has contributed several chapters of this book. Ian was the power that generated this book—as a friend and colleague, his support was valuable for the completion of this book. His persistence and encouragement for moving ahead with the project were the main reasons for its existence.

Several of my teachers, colleagues, and graduate students have contributed mentally to this book. Without them I will not be able to challenge myself for issues to be addressed in this book. My thanks to all of those who challenged me and accepted my extreme ideas. The research team that worked on the United States–Animal Disease Surveillance System (what is currently known as Animal Health Monitoring System) in the early 1980s has contributed to several of the ideas for this book. My thanks and appreciations go to the team members for their input.

Finally, my sincere appreciation goes to my wife Carole Salman, who has been so patient with me in accepting long hours of work. She accepts me as a man attached to veterinary epidemiology.

Mo Salman

Contributors

Laurent Audigé, DVM, PhD
AO Clinical Investigation and Documentation
AO Center
Clavadelerstrasse
CH-7270 Davos Platz
Switzerland
Tel: +41 (44) 200 2462
Fax: +41 (44) 200 2460
e-mail: laurent.audige@ao-asif.ch

Angus Cameron, BVSc, MVS, PhD, MACVSc
AusVet Animal Health Services
140 Falls Road
Wentworth Falls, NSW, 2782
Australia
Tel: +61 2 4757 2770
Fax: +61 2 4757 2789
e-mail: angus@ausvet.com.au

Tim E. Carpenter, MS, PhD
Department of Medicine and Epidemiology
School of Veterinary Medicine
University of California
Davis, California 95616
USA
Tel: +1 530 752 1034
Fax: +1 530 752 0414
e-mail: tecarpenter@ucdavis.edu

Jette Christensen, DVM, PhD
Animal Disease Surveillance,
Canadian Animal Health Network support group
Canadian Food Inspection Agency
93 Mount Edward Road
Charlottetown, Prince Edward Island, C1A 5T1
Canada
Tel: +1 (902) 368 0950 (255)
Fax: +1 (902) 368 0960
e-mail: christensenj@inspection.gc.ca
URL: www.inspection.gc.ca

David A. Dargatz, DVM, MS, PhD, DACT
USDA:APHIS:VS:CEAH
Mail Stop #2E7
2150 Centre Avenue, Building B
Fort Collins, Colorado 80526–8117
USA
Tel: +1 (970) 494 7231
Fax: +1 (970) 494 7228
e-mail: David.A.Dargatz@aphis.usda.gov

Marcus Doherr, DVM, PhD
Division for Clinical Research
Department of Clinical Veterinary Medicine
University of Bern
Bremgartenstrasse 109a
CH-3012 Bern
Switzerland
Tel: +41 (31) 631 2428
Fax: +41 (31) 631 2538
e-mail: marcus.doherr@itn.unibe.ch

Ian Gardner BVSc, MPVM, PhD
Department of Medicine and Epidemiology
School of Veterinary Medicine
University of California
Davis, California 95616
USA
Tel: +1 530 752 6992
Fax: +1 530 752 0414
e-mail: iagardner@ucdavis.edu

Brian J. McCluskey, DVM, MS, PhD, DACVPM
USDA:APHIS:VS:CEAH
Mail Stop #2E7
2150 Centre Avenue, Building B
Fort Collins, Colorado 80526–8117
USA
Tel: +1 (970) 494 7236
Fax: +1 (970) 494 7228
e-mail: Brian.J.Mccluskey@aphis.usda.gov

M.D. (Mo) Salman, BVMS, MPVM, PhD, DACVPM, F.A.C.E.
Animal Population Health Institute
College of Veterinary Medicine and Biomedical Sciences
Colorado State University
Fort Collins, Colorado 80523–1681
USA
Tel: +1 (970) 491–7950
Fax: +1 (970) 491–1889
e-mail: M.D.Salman@colostate.edu

Katharina D.C. Stärk, PhD, Dipl ECVPH
Swiss Federal Veterinary Office
Department of Monitoring
Schwarzenburgstrasse 161
CH-3003 Bern
Switzerland
Tel: +41 31 323 95 44
Fax : +41 31 323 95 43
e-mail: Katharina.Staerk@bvet.admin.ch

Bruce A. Wagner, MS, MA, PhD
USDA:APHIS:VS:CEAH
Mail Stop #2E7
2150 Centre Avenue, Building B
Fort Collins, Colorado 80526–8117
USA
Tel: +1 (970) 494 7256
Fax: +1 (970) 494 7228
e-mail: bruce.a.wagner@aphis.usda.gov

Michael P. Ward, BVSc, MPVM, PhD
Department of Veterinary Pathobiology
School of Veterinary Medicine
Purdue University
West Lafayette, Indiana 47907–2027
USA
Tel: +1 (765) 494–5796
Fax: +1 (765) 494–9830
e-mail: mpw@vet.vet.purdue.edu

Nora E. Wineland, DVM, MS, DACVPM
USDA:APHIS:VS:CEAH
Mail Stop #2E7
2150 Centre Avenue, Building B
Fort Collins, Colorado 80526–8117
USA
Tel: +1 (970) 494 7230
Fax: +1 (970) 494 7228
e-mail: Nora.E.Wineland@aphis.usda.gov

Cristobal Zepeda, DVM, MS
USDA:APHIS:VS:CEAH
Mail Stop #2E7
2150 Centre Avenue, Building B
Fort Collins, Colorado 80526–8117
USA
Tel: +1 (970) 494 7214
Fax: +1 (970) 494 2668
e-mail: Cristobal.Zepeda@usda.gov

ANIMAL DISEASE SURVEILLANCE AND SURVEY SYSTEMS

Methods and Applications

Surveillance and Monitoring Systems for Animal Health Programs and Disease Surveys

M.D. Salman

SURVEILLANCE, MONITORING, AND SURVEYS

DEFINITIONS

Disease monitoring describes the ongoing efforts directed at assessing the health and disease status of a given population. The sampling of individuals from the population to assess disease or health status may be ongoing or repeated. The disease monitored may be a specific infectious disease, a specific production disease, or disease/health in general. The population may be de-

Animal Population Health Institute
College of Veterinary Medicine and Biomedical Sciences
Colorado State University

fined at the national, regional, or herd level. For an alternative definition see Table 1.1.

Disease surveillance is used to describe a more active system and implies that some form of directed action will be taken if the data indicate a disease prevalence or incidence above a certain threshold. Similar to disease monitoring, sampling of individuals from the population to assess disease or health status may be ongoing or repeated, and the population may be defined at the national, regional, or herd level. Surveillance is usually directed at a specific disease. Disease surveillance systems require three components: a defined disease monitoring system, a defined threshold for disease level (predefined critical level at which action will be taken), and predefined directed actions (interventions).

A **disease control program** (DCP) is the combined system of monitoring and surveillance, disease control strategies, and intervention strategies that over a prolonged period of time is employed to reduce the frequency of a specific disease.

A **disease eradication program** (DEP) is a special case of a DCP in which the objective of the program is to eliminate a specific disease (the organism causing the disease).

The term "surveillance" was first used during the French Revolution, when it meant "to keep watch over a group of persons thought to be subversive." The term has been used extensively by epidemiologists and other animal health professionals in the context of monitoring and controlling health-related events in animal populations. Disease surveillance is the key to early warning of a change in the health status of any animal population. It is also essential to provide evidence about the absence of diseases or to determine the extent of a disease that is known to be present. The terms "surveillance" and "monitoring" are often used interchangeably in animal health programs. Animal disease surveillance is watching an animal population closely to determine whether a specific disease or a group of diseases makes an incursion. Monitoring of animal diseases focuses on identifying a disease or a group of diseases to ascertain changes in prevalence and to determine the rate and direction of disease spread. Therefore, by definition, monitoring lacks action to prevent or control a health problem. Surveillance, however, includes an action to prevent or control the health problem that is being monitored. In actual field situations, monitoring usually follows early reaction, should surveillance activities indicate introduction or spread of a disease. Many of the approaches used to implement monitoring can be used for surveillance, and vice versa. In practical terms, the distinction between these two terms often becomes blurred. The differentiation, however, pertains more to the objectives than to the approaches applied.

TABLE 1.1 Definitions of Monitoring and Control Cited in Three Textbooks on Veterinary Epidemiology

Textbook	Definition of monitoring	Surveillance
Martin et al. 1986 Page 259	Animal disease monitoring describes the ongoing efforts directed at assessing the health and disease status of a given population.	The term "disease surveillance" is used to describe a more active system and implies that some form of directed action will be taken if the data indicate a disease level above a certain threshold.
Thrusfield 1995 Page 22	Monitoring is the making of routine observations on health, productivity, and environmental factors and the recording and transmission of these observations.	Surveillance is a more intensive form of data recording than monitoring.
Pages 358, 360	The routine collection of information on disease, productivity, and other characteristics possibly related to them in a population.	An intensive form of monitoring (q.v.). Designed so that action can be taken to improve the health status of a population; therefore, it is frequently used in disease control campaigns.
Noordhuizen et al. 1997 Page 379	Monitoring refers to a continuous, dynamic process of collecting data about health and disease and their determinants in a given population over a defined time period (descriptive epidemiology).	Surveillance refers to a specific extension of monitoring where obtained information is used and measures are taken if certain threshold values related to disease status have been passed. It, therefore, is part of disease control programs.

The term "survey" is used to indicate an investigation or a study in which information is systematically collected for a specific aim or conceptual hypothesis. The time frame for this type of investigation is a specific and usually short period of time. This is in contrast to surveillance and monitoring, which involve the ongoing systematic collection of data and information. Surveys are more frequently used to answer a specific research question oriented toward a scientific and exploratory purpose. Approaches used for survey studies are similar to those used for surveillance and monitoring. In concept, a series of surveys can be considered as a monitoring system that may transition into a surveillance system if action is taken to prevent or control the disease. Therefore, the terms "surveillance," "monitoring," and "survey" share several common components, and hence, it is logical to consider them as a single topic for the purpose of this book.

Some authors have proposed the use of the term "monitoring and surveillance system" (MOSS) to summarize the concepts and approaches (Doherr and Audigé 2001; Noordhuizen et al. 1997; Stärk 1996). In that context, monitoring describes a continuous, adaptable process of collecting data about diseases and their determinants in a given population, but without any immediate control activities. Surveillance is a specific case of monitoring in which control or eradication measures are implemented whenever certain threshold levels related to the infection or disease status have been exceeded. By definition, surveillance is therefore part of any disease control program (Noordhuisen et al. 1997; Office International des Epizooties [OIE] 1998, 2000). The term "MOSS" will be used hereafter in this book, and surveys are included in this term unless otherwise mentioned.

DATA COLLECTION METHOD FOR MOSS

One of the main components for any MOSS is the collection of data, which can be classified as either passive or active. Unfortunately, some authors have generalized these terms as labeling surveillance as passive versus active (Lilienfeld and Stolley 1994). A surveillance system cannot be passive if an action is part of its definition. Therefore, in this book the use of the terms "active" and "passive" will be only used to refer to the data collection method.

An active collection of data for a MOSS is referred to as the systematic or regular recording of cases of a designated disease or a group of diseases for a specific goal of monitoring or surveillance. A population determined by specific location or time period is usually defined for the system. This should provide each individual within the defined population with a known and often equal chance of being selected. The identification of such an appropriate population depends on the event of interest, its expected prevalence, and the available diagnostic tests. Another chapter (Chapter 4) of this book details the sampling techniques for this type of MOSS.

Information about the health-related event might be collected from owners by interview or mail. Biological samples might be collected during farm visits or at abattoirs, knackeries, or carcass rendering plants. In addition, the screening of animal medical records (either the files or electronic databases) for specific entries or the screening of biological sample banks for specific pathogens or lesions can be considered part of the active collection of data for a MOSS. Examples of such a system include the tuberculosis and brucellosis MOSSs that are routinely performed in several countries of the world, infectious bovine rhinotracheitis (IBR) and enzootic bovine leucosis (EBL) sero-surveys in Switzerland (Stärk 1996), abattoir screening for contagious bovine pleuropneumonia (CBPP) in Switzerland (Stärk 1996), bovine spongiform encephalopathy (BSE) screening of fallen stock and emergency slaughtered cattle in Switzerland and Europe (Doherr et al. 1999, 2001) and of "downer cows" in the United States (http://www.aphis.usda.gov/lpa/issues/bse/bse.html). Other examples would be the scrapie surveillance in the United Kingdom (Simmons et al. 2000) and postal surveys for scrapie in the United Kingdom, the Netherlands, and Switzerland (Baumgarten et al. 2002; Hoinville et al. 1999, 2000; Morgan et al. 1990; Schreuder et al. 1993). Some national MOSSs include mail or interview questionnaires as well as collection of biological samples for laboratory testing (Kane et al. 2000; Traub-Dargatz et al. 2000a, 2000b; Wagner et al. 2000).

A major disadvantage of the active data collection for a MOSS, when population-based, is that it is very costly when the occurrence of the target disease is rare. The lower the disease prevalence, the larger the sample size required for detection. Once the prevalence becomes very low ($<0.1\%$), it often is not feasible to further increase the sample size because of funding constraints, because of limitations in the working capacity of diagnostic laboratories, or simply because of limitations of the chosen test system (e.g., the tests are not sensitive and specific enough to distinguish between zero and very low prevalence levels). The situation changes from low prevalence to the probability of disease freedom. Instead of prevalence estimation, the focus is now on the identification of a health-related event if it occurs in the defined population above the threshold prevalence. An example in which all animals in a defined population are tested is the mandatory fallen stock surveillance for BSE in Europe. Within this program, because of the expected very low prevalence ($<0.1\%$) of detectable cases, all fallen cattle more than 24 months of age have to be examined. Between January 2001 and April 2002, the average prevalence in this high-risk target population was approximately 0.05%—or one case per 2,000 samples tested (http://europa.eu.int/comm/food/fs/bse/testing/bse _results_en.html).

The passive collection of data involves the reporting of clinical or subclinical suspect cases to the health authorities by health care professionals, at their discretion (Lilienfeld and Stolley 1994). Therefore, the validity of the system depends solely on the willingness of these professionals to secure the flow of data. In veterinary medicine, the passive collection of data can be influenced by the awareness and level of knowledge of a particular disease among veterinary practitioners and producers or owners of animals. Another important component of this type of data collection is the availability of a diagnostic laboratory scheme to support and confirm cases. The main limitation of passive data collection is inconsistency in the data collection for different diseases and among communities that provide the data. Thus, a comparison of various passively collected MOSS data should be approached with caution. Disease awareness, educational level of the MOSS data providers (practitioners, regulatory veterinarians, and owners/producers), and the nature of the disease under the MOSS are the major elements in the effectiveness of the MOSS. For instance, a disease with a high case-fatality rate may be reported more frequently than a disease with a low case-fatality rate. A disease with more public awareness (e.g., one that has had extensive advertising or educational programs) may be more likely to be reported compared with a disease with less awareness, even though its true prevalence and incidence are lower. It should be also noted that the use of the passive collection of data would not ensure the early detection of a disease.

Passive collection of data for a MOSS can identify a change in a pattern that may warrant further investigation. Typically, an active method of collection of data then can be implemented. For instance, the first few BSE cases found in the United Kingdom at the initial epidemic were reported using the passive collection of data for a MOSS that was not designed specifically for collection of BSE cases. Then a MOSS was implemented to actively collect data for BSE.

Some countries have used the term "notifiable animal diseases" for those diseases that are required by law to be reported. Most of the OIE List A and specific zoonotic diseases fit the criteria to be on the notifiable list. Although these notifiable diseases by definition should require active collection of data for a MOSS, most countries have used passive collection of data for MOSSs. The main reason for this is the lack of a well-planned study design to maintain and actively detect cases for these diseases.

Other authors (Doherr and Audigé 2001; Dufour and Audigé 1997) have classified MOSS activities by the method of data collection into three classes: passive, active, and sentinel networks. Baseline data collection was considered a subcategory of passive collection. In my opinion, a disease trend that is determined by surveillance is different from baseline data. Disease trends can change over time, and the use of the term "baseline data" in this context may be misleading. The term "sentinel networks" refers to a method for actively collecting data for a MOSS using a selected sample to represent the population. Chapter 8 discusses details of the use of sentinel herds for MOSSs.

TARGETED SURVEILLANCE

The term "targeted surveillance" is becoming popular, and it principally refers to focusing the sampling for the MOSS on high-risk populations (i.e., targeted populations) in which specific commonly known risk factors exist. An example of a target population is fallen cattle stock in Europe, because this high-risk group of cattle has more BSE than otherwise healthy cattle. Another target population is specific hamburger meat processed in large quantities, which is associated with a greater risk of *Escherichia coli* O157:H7 than unprocessed meat.

The main purpose of implementing this surveillance approach is to increase the efficiency of the system. This design is appropriate when the following two conditions exist: the disease under consideration is less common in the general population than in the targeted group, and specific risk factors are established or known. Therefore, prior knowledge about the disease and its epidemiology is required before this design can be considered. On occasion, targeted surveillance is used to ensure the absence of a specific disease from a highly susceptible population. For instance, the purpose of the surveillance in the United States of downer cows and cattle with suspected neurological signs of BSE is mainly to provide evidence of the absence of BSE.

Targeted surveillance is an effective design to purposely implement an action that can reduce the effect of a disease rapidly. An example of this approach is a nosocomial infection MOSS in a veterinary teaching hospital in which equine colic cases are targeted for *Salmonella* surveillance. This is because of the fact that these cases are more susceptible to this infection than other hospital-admitted cases (Kim et al. 2001; Tillotson et al. 1997).

EFFECT OF THE CHANGE IN TRADE REGULATIONS ON MOSS PLANNING AND IMPLEMENTATION

Among the agreements that were included in the treaty that established the World Trade Organization (WTO) is the Agreement on the Application of Sanitary and Phytosanitary Measures (SPS) Agreement, which sets out the basic rules for food safety and animal and plant health standards. The SPS Agreement has truly changed the way in which trade decisions related to agricultural products are made. Its main intent is to avoid the use of SPS measures as unjustified barriers to trade. Although recognizing the right of countries to protect human health and agricultural health, the agreement dictates that all measures must be scientifically based and not unnecessarily restrictive. Specifically, the SPS agreement has placed an increased emphasis on the importance of sanitary and phytosanitary measures, requiring improved surveillance and monitoring systems, adequate laboratory diagnosis, risk analysis capabilities, and quality assurance. The agreement demands that a country demonstrate its animal health status by means of scientifically based surveillance efforts. Thus, a country's veterinary services, livestock industries, and international agencies are paying attention to the design, implementation, and outcomes of MOSSs for animal diseases in both animals and animal products (Zepeda et al. 2001).

In several countries, the demand for scientifically reliable MOSS has coincided with a reduction in budgetary and human resources among the government veterinary services. These countries, therefore, have attempted to identify the most efficient methods to satisfy the national and international requirements for animal health. During the last decade, numerous methods and approaches for MOSS in animal health programs have been discussed or proposed. The most important outcome from this type of exploration is the determination of the absence of the disease or its agent from a country; that is, when prevalence of a disease is at or near zero. The objective of this type of MOSS is to provide evidence (with known confidence) that a disease or pathogen, if present in a zone or country, is present at or below an acceptably low (practically undetectable) prevalence. Although it will probably continue to be commonly used, the term "freedom from disease" is potentially misleading. Freedom implies complete absence, which is analogous to the now unacceptable concept of zero risk.

Current approaches generally involve the compilation of evidence from a range of sources and the use of this evidence to put forward a convincing argument about a country's disease status. One source of evidence that is commonly used or demanded is a structured statistically valid survey. The primary advantages of the use of surveys are that well-established theory and methodologies exist and that they are able to produce a quantifiable probability estimate for the presence of disease. International regulations increasingly demand that the level of proof of disease status meets quantitative standards; for example, that the probability of the presence of disease at a prevalence in animals of 0.2% or greater is less than 1%. Other sources of evidence that may be used include passively collected data, an assessment of the quality of the veterinary services, livestock movement history, geographical and environmental factors, abattoir monitoring, sentinel herds, and so forth.

It has become clear that there are a number of problems with this approach. Structured surveys are often too expensive or impractical to achieve the level of proof required. This is a result of the very large sample sizes necessary when the prevalence is very low and when applied tests do not have very high sensitivity and specificity. This difficulty is further complicated by variability in sensitivity and specificity and by a lack of reliable estimates of these test accuracy parameters for the population under study.

As a result, true disease status cannot always be determined through the use of surveys alone. It is necessary to combine all the different sources of evidence available to assess the overall probability that a disease does not exist or is below the threshold prevalence. Until now, however, there have been no accepted methodologies for either quantifying the evidence provided by passive collection of data for a MOSS or combining probability estimates from multiple different sources into an overall estimate of the probability of absence of the disease. It is proposed that these problems may now be overcome through the use of a range of different analytical methods, including

- a standardized approach to scenario tree analysis and stochastic simulation to estimate the power of a complex MOSS (A. Cameron, personal communication),
- improved use of techniques to elicit and combine expert opinion as additional information to data generated by a MOSS (K. Stärk, personal communication),
- methods to adjust the value of data sources for a MOSS based on the time that has passed since their generation (Schlosser and Ebel 2001),
- and Bayesian approaches to the combination of data from multiple sources of MOSS (Suess et al. 2002).

Regardless of whether one or a combination of the above approaches is used, there is a need to ensure that the principles behind it, and the tools required to implement it, are sound and made widely available to those who need it. The use of these approaches would require specific tasks:

1. Identify all possible sources of evidence for the absence of disease.
2. Analyze each source independently through the construction of a scenario tree to estimate the probability that an infected animal, if present, would be identified by the MOSS. At each branch of the tree, probability estimates and ranges are required. These should be derived from reliable

data sources, if available, or from formally structured expert opinion methods if no reliable data are available.

3. Use stochastic methods to determine a point estimate of the probability of detecting disease based on a scenario tree, as well as the probability distribution around that estimate (to provide measures of confidence).
4. Adjust all values for the time elapsed since data collection.
5. Combine the estimates from all different sources of evidence to provide an overall probability and confidence level.
6. If the resultant probability is inadequate to meet international standards, either use sensitivity analysis to determine which method may be most effective at increasing the level of confidence or conduct a (relatively small) structured survey to fill the probability gap.

Chapters 4, 5, 6, and 7 of this book elaborate on these methods and their application. Although there are limited examples of application of some of these approaches, there are also many countries struggling to adjust to the new world trade environment. A significant effort needs to be initiated by governments and international organizations to achieve compliance with the SPS Agreement in terms of the demonstration of absence of a disease. International funding organizations need to adjust their policies and be willing to support the development of sustainable infrastructures that will allow countries access to the world marketplace.

BIBLIOGRAPHY

Baumgarten L., Heim D., Fatzer R., Zurbriggen A., Doherr M.G. 2002. Assessment of the Swiss approach to scrapie surveillance. Vet Rec 151(18):545–547.

Doherr M.G., Audigé L. 2001. Monitoring and surveillance for rare health-related events—A review from the veterinary perspective. Phil Trans R Soc Lond B 356:1097–1106.

Doherr M.G., Oesch B., Moser B., Vandevelde M., Heim D. 1999. Targeted surveillance for bovine spongiform encephalopathy (BSE). Vet Rec 145:672.

Doherr M.G., Heim D., Fatzer R., Cohen C.H., Vandevelde M., Zurbriggen A. 2001. Targeted screening of high-risk cattle populations for BSE to augment mandatory reporting of clinical suspects. Prev Vet Med 51:3–16.

Dufour B., Audigé L. 1997. A proposed classification of veterinary epidemiosurveillance networks. Rev Sci Technol Off Int Epiz 16:746–758.

Hoinville L., McLean A.R., Hoek A., Gravenor M.B., Wilesmith J. 1999. Scrapie occurrence in Great Britain. Vet Rec 145:405–406.

Hoinville L.J., Hoek A., Gravenor M.B., McLean, A.R. 2000. Descriptive epidemiology of scrapie in Great Britain: Results of a postal survey. Vet Rec 146(16):455–461.

Kane A.J., Traub-Dargatz J.L., Losinger W.C., Garber L.P., Wagner B.A., Hill G.W. 2000. A cross-sectional study of lameness and lamenitis in U.S. horses. Proceeding abstract 441. Ninth Meeting of the International Society of Veterinary Epidemiology and Economics. August 6–12, 2000, Breckenridge, Colorado.

Kim, L.M., Morley, P.S., Traub-Dargatz, J.L., Salman, M.D., Gentry-Weeks, C. 2001. Factors associated with *Salmonella* shedding among equine colic patients at a veterinary teaching hospital. J Am Vet Med Assoc 218(5):740–748.

Lilienfeld D.E., Stolley P.D., Eds. 1994. Foundations of Epidemiology, 3rd ed. Oxford University Press, New York.

Martin S.W., Meek A.H., Willeberg P. 1986. Veterinary epidemiology. Principles and methods. Iowa State University Press, Ames.

Morgan K.L., Nicholas K., Glover M.J., Hall A.P. 1990. A questionnaire survey of the prevalence of scrapie in sheep in Britain. Vet Rec 127:373–376.

Noordhuizen J.P.T.M., Frankena K., van der Hoofd C.M., Graat E.A.M., Eds. 1997. Application of quantitative methods in veterinary epidemiology. Wageningen Press, Wageningen, The Netherlands.

Office International des Epizooties. 1998. Guide to epidemiological surveillance for rinderpest. Rev Sci Technol Off Int Epiz 17(3):796–824.

Office International des Epizooties. 2000. Recommended standard for epidemiological surveillance systems for rinderpest. Office International des Epizooties, International Animal Health Code Part 3, Section 3.8, Appendix 3.8.1.

Schlosser W., Ebel E.D. 2001. Use of a Markov-chain Monte Carlo model to evaluate the time value of historical testing information in animal populations. Prev Vet Med 48:167–175.

Schreuder B.E.C., de Jong M.C.M., Pekelder J.J., Vellema P., Broker A.J.M., Betcke H. 1993. Prevalence and incidence of scrapie in the Netherlands: A questionnaire survey. Vet Rec 133:211–14.

Simmons M.M., Ryder S.J., Chaplin M.C., Spencer Y.I., Webb C.R., Hoinville L.J., Ryan J., Stack M.J., Wells G.A., Wilesmith J.W. 2000. Scrapie surveillance in Great Britain: Results of an abattoir survey, 1997/98. Vet Rec 146(14):391–395.

Stärk K.D. 1996 Animal health monitoring and surveillance in Switzerland. Aust Vet J 73(3):96–97.

Suess, E.A., Gardner, I.A., Johnson, W.O. 2002. Hierarchical Bayesian model for prevalence inferences and determination of a country's status for an animal disease. Prev Vet Med 55:155–171.

Thrusfield M. 1995. Veterinary epidemiology. Blackwell Science, Oxford.

Tillotson K., Savage C.J., Salman M.D., Gentry-Weeks C.R., Rice D., Fedorka-Cray P.J., Hendrickson D.A., Jones R.L., Nelson A.W., Traub-Dargatz J.L. 1997. An outbreak of *Salmonella infantis* infection in a large animal veterinary teaching hospital. J Am Vet Med Assoc 211:1554–1557.

Traub-Dargatz J.L., Garber L.P., Hill G.W., Wagner B.A., Losinger W.C., Seitzinger A.H., Rodriguez J.M., Stanton N.G. 2000a. Overview of the initial phase of the National Animal Health Monitoring Systems (NAHMS) equine '98 study. Proceeding abstract 64. Ninth Meeting of the International Society of Veterinary Epidemiology and Economics. August 6–12, 2000, Breckenridge, Colorado.

Traub-Dargatz J.L., Garber L.P., Fedorka-Cray P.J., Ladely S., Ferris K.E. 2000b. Fecal shedding of *Salmonella* spp. by horses in the United States during 1998 and 1999 and detection of *Salmonella* spp. in grain and concentrate sources on equine operations. J Am Vet Med Assoc 217(2):226–230.

Wagner B.A., Wise D.J., Khoo L.H. 2000. Health monitoring in the U.S. catfish industry. Proceeding abstract 358. Ninth Meeting of the International Society of Veterinary Epidemiology and Economics. August 6–12, 2000, Breckenridge, Colorado.

Zepeda C., Salman M.D., Ruppanner R. 2001. International trade, animal health, and veterinary epidemiology: Challenge and opportunities. Prev Vet Med 48:261–272.

Application of Surveillance and Monitoring Systems in Disease Control Programs

J. Christensen

INTRODUCTION

This chapter describes the application of monitoring and surveillance systems (MOSSs) in disease control and disease eradication programs by introduction of a disease control model. This model introduces the concept that disease control is a process.

In addition to monitoring and surveillance, this chapter presents control measures and intervention strategies as the basis for disease control or eradication programs. It will discuss circumstances that influence decisions made in the disease control process. They may affect the design of monitoring and surveillance and, therefore, the disease control or eradication program. The scope describes the process of disease control programs at the national (or regional)

Canadian Food Inspection Agency
Charlottetown
Prince Edward Island
Canada

level, not specifically in individual herds. Some aspects may apply equally well to the herd level, but the reader will need to make the extrapolation. Therefore, unless stated otherwise, the following circumstances will be assumed throughout this chapter: Population: the national herd of an animal species; disease: foreign animal disease (FAD; e.g., Office International des Epizooties [OIE] list A or B diseases [http://www.oie.int/] or other undesired diseases unwanted in a country or region).

MODEL

In this section, the MOSS will link the system with disease control or eradication programs; this section also discusses the dynamics of a disease control program (DCP). A visual model is introduced to present the concept that disease control is a process.

BASELINE SET UP AND ASSUMPTIONS

The disease is a specific infectious disease, for example, FAD, as the OIE list A and B diseases, or an emerging disease. Further, it is assumed the disease has never been introduced into the population or, if it has been introduced, that it has not been present for many years. The population is all animals of all relevant species in a country (or a region). The host range of the disease determines the relevance of an animal species.

Some examples of disease and population are foot and mouth disease (FMD) in the United Kingdom in 2001 (an example of a FAD; http://europa.eu .int/comm/food/fs/ah_pcad/ah_pcad_47_en.pdf), with a population of all susceptible animals in the United Kingdom (cows, sheep, goats, pigs, etc.), and porcine reproductive and respiratory syndrome (PRRS) in the 1990s, with a population of all pigs in any European country.

The disease control model would not apply to production diseases with multiple causative agents; for example, mastitis, in which the model was not developed for the situation where the individual herd is the population. However, if relevant, with few alterations, the model might describe the process from introduction of a new disease to its eradication, when the population is the herd.

DISEASE CONTROL MODEL

In the disease control model (Christensen 2001), there are three columns: type of monitoring, disease status, and activity (Figure 2.1). Time is not a component of the model; therefore, none of the three columns indicates the length of the periods throughout the process. Starting at the top of Figure 2.1, the pop-

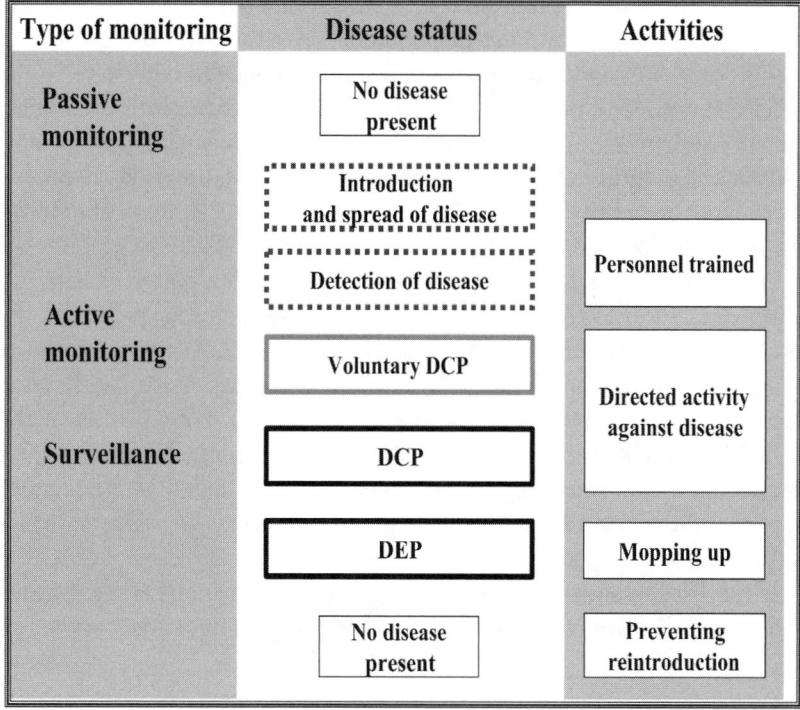

FIGURE 2.1   The disease control model. A visual model describing a disease control or eradication process from introduction of disease (foreign animal disease or an emerging disease) to eradication.

ulation is free of disease and the level of expertise available to diagnose and control the disease would be totally dependent on the quality of the FAD preparedness work plan of the country.

In countries in which a specific infectious disease has never been present or the last outbreak is dated generations ago (e.g. rinderpest in Northern Europe), there would be few or no professional people—farmers or veterinarians—with personal experience of the clinical signs of this disease. In addition, the diagnostic laboratories would have very little experience in the appropriate diagnostic tools. Therefore, if maintaining adequate expertise and diagnostic facilities is not part of the FAD preparedness, very little or no expertise to diagnose or control will be available in the event of an outbreak.

At some point, the disease may be introduced into the population from other countries or other animal species or recur because existing agents have mutated. After this introduction, the agent (e.g., a parasite, bacterium, virus, or prion) may start to spread among animals in infected and uninfected herds.

At first the introduction and spread of disease may be undetected (or not reported), and time to detection depends on the severity of clinical signs including the mortality and adverse effects on production, the morbidity in the affected herds, the familiarity of farmers and veterinarians with the clinical signs of the disease, and the speed the disease spreads among herds. High mortality and high morbidity, as is evident when Aujeszky's disease is introduced into a fully susceptible herd with piglets, tend to be detected soon after introduction (Figure 2.2). In contrast, sporadic diseases, for which the problem is a human health risk, may take years to detect. For example, bovine spongiform encephalopathy (BSE) in cattle tends to have a delayed detection because of the low level of infection between and among herds, morbidity, and similarities of its symptoms with other diseases. Although fatal, the disease is sporadic in affected herds. An additional complication to early detection of BSE is that in the beginning, the clinical signs are not associated with a notifiable disease. Even though the mortality among clinically affected cows is high, BSE is not a production-limiting disease and, therefore, was only detected as a problem when it was suspected to be a human health risk.

In the disease control structure model, there is a distinction between passive and active collection of data for a MOSS. This distinction between active and

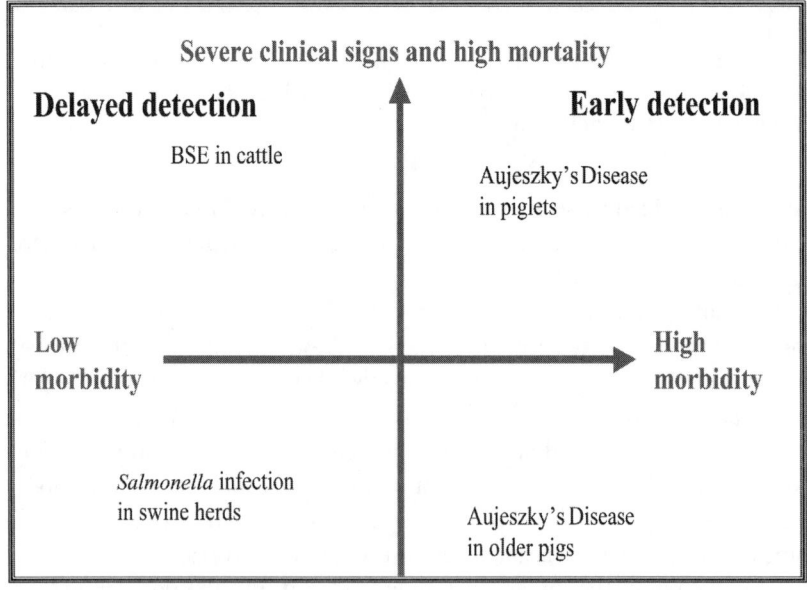

FIGURE 2.2   Detection of a foreign animal disease depends on severity of the disease and morbidity. Lack of knowledge of the disease tends to shift detection toward the lower-left quadrant.

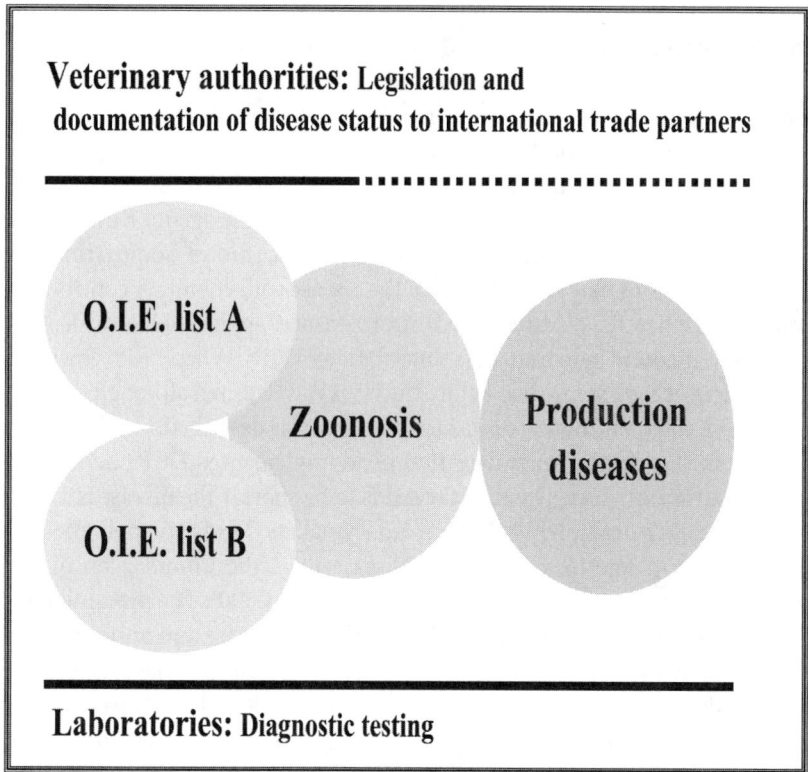

Veterinary authorities: Legislation and documentation of disease status to international trade partners

O.I.E. list A

Zoonosis

Production diseases

O.I.E. list B

Laboratories: Diagnostic testing

FIGURE 2.3   Unique roles of the veterinary authorities and laboratories in national disease control and disease eradication programs. Legislation rests with the veterinary authorities (upper solid line). Documentation of disease status may or may not rest with the veterinary authorities (upper dashed line). Laboratories will be responsible for diagnostic tests (lower solid line).

passive collection of data (Figure 2.3) may be a bit controversial but is useful in the understanding of this structure model. It is usual for systematic sampling and diagnostic testing for the specific disease to be done until a disease has been detected as a problem in a population. Therefore, there is no active monitoring of the disease. However, the general awareness of clinical disease is a passive collection of data for monitoring of the population for new diseases and clinical signs (e.g., abortions or preweaning mortality may cause detection of a disease like Aujeszky's disease or PRRS).

The monitoring may become active and retraining of personnel may be initiated when the disease is detected and researchers, veterinarians (government, industry, and private), and farmers attempt to gain more knowledge about the disease. They assess the magnitude of the problem regardless of whether it is economically important or is linked with a human health risk.

If the disease is a well-known FAD (e.g., OIE list A), detection will result in immediate action to control or eradicate the disease, and laboratory staff, veterinary practitioners, and farmers are retrained to detect clinical signs, to diagnose, and to treat the disease.

For emerging diseases, the pathogenesis and etiologic agent of the disease may be investigated in experiments or epidemiologic studies. Some farmers or their organizations may start to combat the disease with voluntary control programs. Therefore, the research and control measures applied will provide valuable knowledge and help train personnel for later DCPs. When PRRS emerged, for example, it took some time before the virus was detected although the clinical disease (blue ear disease or mystery disease) was described.

The time lag from disease detection to an implemented DCP (Δt) may be long or extremely short. The time lag tends to be short if the disease is a well-known FAD, for example, FMD; or if policymakers decide to apply the precautionary principle to an emerging disease (e.g., the Commission of the European Communities policy for BSE; Anonymous 2000). The precautionary principle is usually derived from both scientific knowledge and public perception information. Application of the precautionary principle may result in the political decision to eliminate the disease by proceeding directly to a disease eradication program (DEP). Policymakers apply this precautionary principle if they are faced with an unacceptable risk, scientific uncertainty, public concerns, or a combination of all three. Application of the precautionary principle may result in the political decision to eliminate the disease by proceeding directly to a DEP.

The time lag tends to be longer when there is uncertainty about prevalence, the speed of the disease spread (i.e., its incidence), validity of the diagnostic and screening tests, how rapidly the disease will spread, and appropriate interventions, especially if the FAD disease is not a threat to human health and the economic effect is manageable.

In a DCP or DEP, specific components to be implemented in a MOSS directed against the disease are

- monitoring is targeted at the disease,
- thresholds for interventions against the disease are defined,
- predefined interventions are implemented to reduce disease occurrence,
- the total population (all herds in the country) is included,
- and legislative measures may be necessary to ensure the inclusion of the entire herd population.

The ultimate aim of a DCP for a FAD is often its later evolution into a DEP. This also depends on the circumstances; that is, it is most successful when the prevalence is low and eradication is an option. The effort to detect the last case can be intensive, and testing the population that most likely is to be freed from the disease usually is the end point of the DEP (cleaning up).

At the end of a successful DEP, no disease is present in the country, and the only activities are to prevent reintroduction and, ideally, the maintenance of a limited MOSS specifically to prevent reintroduction of the disease, limit the spread of the disease after an introduction, and document freedom from disease. If the FAD is not reintroduced, the country will eventually return to the top of the model again (i.e., the starting point).

In conclusion, the disease control model describes the MOSS and activities from before an outbreak until eradication is achieved as a disease control process.

ESSENTIAL BUILDING MATERIALS FOR DCPs

A portion of the MOSS is the control strategies, which are the building materials for the DCP. An important message that the disease control model can communicate is that control and intervention strategies will adapt to changing circumstances.

CONTROL STRATEGY

The control strategy describes the aim of the actions (i.e., efforts or measures) taken against disease, and they can be classified as

- **Prevention**, applied to those measures designed to exclude disease from an unaffected population.
- **Control**, associated with the efforts directed toward reducing the frequency of existing disease to levels biologically or economically justifiable or otherwise of little consequence.
- **Eradication**, describing the efforts to eliminate selected organisms from a defined population. Animal species and location (herd, region, or country) define the population.

There is one more strategy, **inactivity**, but this strategy is only applicable when for biological, political, economic, cultural, or social reasons it is decided not to take action against a specific disease.

TABLE 2.1   Interventions and Strategy

Type of intervention	Aims at control strategy
Slaughter	
Stamping out	Eradication
Depopulation/repopulation	Eradication
Test and slaughter	Reduction
Culling	Reduction
Reduction of contact	
Quarantine	Prevention
Movement restrictions	Prevention
All-in all-out (batch production)	Prevention
Chemical use	
Preventive or strategic treatment	Prevention
Therapeutic treatment	Reduction
Disinfection	Reduction
Pesticides	Reduction
Modification of host resistance	
Vaccination	Prevention
Genetic resistance	Prevention
Environment and or management control	
Improved husbandry	Prevention or reduction
Feeding	Prevention or reduction
Education	Prevention or reduction
Biological control	Prevention or reduction
Doing nothing	

Note. One or more interventions can be combined in an intervention strategy. For example, multiple interventions have been applied in the Danish Salmonella Control Program (Chapter 12).

INTERVENTION STRATEGIES

Actions directed against disease are intervention measures (Table 2.1). Most of these measures are well-known tools used in practice to cure disease or control diseases in herds. Sometimes the term intervention strategy is used for a combination of intervention measures.

CIRCUMSTANCES INFLUENCING DECISIONS IN THE DCP

It has been alluded that in the disease control process, circumstances influence the decisions regarding monitoring, control, and the intervention strategy. Even before introduction of disease, circumstances may influence decisions. An example is the focus and efforts to improve the FAD preparedness plan in many countries following the 2001 outbreak of FMD in the United Kingdom.

In general, the circumstances are related to

Nature of the disease
- The disease
- Disease characteristics in populations
- Treatment and interventions

People
- Political issues
- Economic considerations
- Cultural or social factors

Infrastructure
- Veterinary authorities
- Diagnostic laboratories
- Livestock industries

Information
- Science-based
- Other

NATURE OF THE DISEASE

The nature of the disease is pivotal for the decisions in the initial phases of an outbreak of FAD throughout the control and eradication campaign and even when no disease is present.

To describe the "nature of the disease," we need to understand the processes of the disease: cause, pathogenesis, transmission of disease among individuals and among populations, treatment, and so forth. A full description of all components that will describe the nature of disease is beyond the scope of this book. Here, some key components that may influence decisions on MOSSs, DCPs, and DEPs are mentioned as examples.

Disease Cause

If the disease has one necessary cause or an etiologic agent (e.g., specific infectious disease) or if it is multifactorial, this will determine the control strategy of the program (DCP or DEP). A MOSS is not usually directly influenced.

FAD, as in the OIE list A and B diseases, and zoonoses are specific infectious diseases with one necessary cause, be it a prion, virus, bacterium, or parasite. Therefore, DEPs and DCPs are feasible and have been adopted in many countries to combat OIE list A and B diseases.

Even for production-limiting diseases that are typically multifactorial (e.g., mastitis), DCPs have been adopted. However, an elimination strategy for mastitis in a dairy farm would imply elimination of all combinations of adverse factors (sufficient causes) that cause mastitis. This elimination of sufficient causes is impossible, and therefore, a DEP is not feasible. What would be achievable however, is a DEP for one specific mastitis agent in the herd; for example, *Staphylococcus aureus* infection.

Host Range and Survival in the Environment

For a specific causative agent, host range (main host species, vectors, intermediate hosts, etc.) and survival in the environment will influence the applicable methods of a MOSS and its control or intervention strategy.

For a DCP to be effective, the MOSS should include all susceptible animal species that may have contact with the population of interest. For example, a DEP for FMD should consider all cloven-hoofed animals in the country (cattle, sheep, pigs, cloven-hoofed zoo animals and wildlife, etc.). Another complication to a DCP/DEP may be infected wildlife reservoirs that can potentially have contact with domestic animals in the population of interest. Bovine tuberculosis (TB) in badgers (Martin et al. 1997) and possums (Paterson and Morris 1995) poses a threat to the cattle populations in the United Kingdom, the Republic of Ireland, and New Zealand.

A wide host range and prolonged survival of the infective agent in the environment might even influence the feasibility of a DCP/DEP. For example, it may be impossible to eradicate TB from the cattle population in the United Kingdom, the Republic of Ireland, or New Zealand if the agent cannot be eliminated from the herd environment (pasture) and contact to the infected wildlife cannot be avoided.

Host-agent Interaction

The interaction between host and agent influences the possibilities for MOSS and, therefore, the feasibility of a DCP or DEP.

Clinical signs usually are the first manifestation of the disease; therefore, specific clinical signs are important for early detection of disease, especially if the transmission of disease is rapid. Subtle or ambiguous clinical signs, subclinical disease, and presence of healthy carriers impede early detection, and monitoring or surveillance will have to rely on other methods.

A strong specific antibody response of the host is often the key element in monitoring specific diseases because serologic methods generally are suitable for large-scale testing (which is economically and practically efficient), in contrast to antigen detection (which is often time-consuming and labor intensive).

Transmission

Knowledge of the transmission potential chain (e.g., excretion, mode of transmission, mechanism of entry, susceptibility of the potential host) can help a MOSS at a target or sentinel population. The transmission chain may also influence the prevention of disease.

The transmission mode can be vertical, horizontal, direct, or indirect, and specific diseases may have one primary mode of transmission. For infectious disease, direct animal-to-animal contact (horizontal) usually plays a key role in spread of disease, and hence, trade and movement restrictions have been a cornerstone in FAD control.

Diagnostic Methods

A MOSS requires large-scale diagnostic testing; therefore, fast, inexpensive, and accurate diagnostic tests will be preferred. The implications of the accuracy of the diagnostic test on monitoring are discussed in Chapters 4 and 5. Following are some practical considerations that influence monitoring.

The diagnostic test will determine which material (feces, blood, brain, etc.), the amount of this material, and the method of shipment to laboratories. These factors will have an effect on the large-scale collection of samples because both the availability of samples and the ease of collection are influenced. The cost and rapidity of the diagnostic test will also influence the effectiveness of monitoring.

DISEASE CHARACTERISTICS IN POPULATIONS

Morbidity and mortality are measured in the disease monitoring as true prevalence or incidence rates, and decisions about a DCP/DEP depend, to a certain extent, on knowledge of morbidity and mortality.

Morbidity and mortality influence early detection of the disease at both the national level and the herd level. This can have an effect on the number of infected herds and animals when the disease is first detected. Within-herd morbidity and mortality will have an effect on the herd-level diagnostic test performance (see Chapters 4 and 5). Morbidity, and possibly mortality, will also have an effect on total cost of the remaining DCP/DEP; therefore, the progress of a DCP/DEP may be measured by changes in morbidity or mortality.

TREATMENT AND INTERVENTION

Treatment and intervention methods have no influence on the MOSS; however, predefined intervention is part of the system. Therefore, a MOSS without intervention is contradictory, and a DCP/DEP without intervention is contradictory.

Therapeutic measures or preventive treatment of individual animals or groups are interventions that usually involve chemical use (Table 2.1). Therapeutic treatment and vaccination of individuals may be applicable for some bacterial and parasitic diseases. For viral infections, however, therapeutic treatment is generally not applicable, and vaccination may be the only option if an effective vaccine is available. Some diseases, for example, prion diseases, are untreatable. For these diseases, when no individual animal treatment is available, herd-level interventions may be applied (Table 2.1).

In summary, in Table 2.2 are found two profiles of specific infectious diseases with a nature that will either facilitate a successful DEP or make the DEP complex or impossible and, thus, make acceptance of the DCP the best option.

In general, specific infectious diseases, as are most FADs, have a nature somewhere between the two extremes, which can make decisions difficult. Therefore, additional circumstances will influence the decisions about MOSSs in general and the DCP/DEP in specific.

PEOPLE

Issues relating to people influence decisions about MOSS in animal populations or their products. Some MOSSs are primarily for the benefit of human health; for example, meat inspection is a MOSS to ensure food safety and quality. A DCP/DEP for zoonosis (TB, brucellosis, BSE, *Salmonella*, etc.) is motivated by human health more than by the health and production effect on animals. Even some of the OIE list A and B diseases are defined as those with a serious socioeconomic or public health consequence. (http://www.oie.int/).

TABLE 2.2   Profiles of Two Specific Infectious Diseases

Disease 1	Disease 2
A narrow host range (one animal species), no vectors or intermediate hosts	A wide host range (may be including wildlife, vectors and intermediate hosts
Few well-known transmission modes (e.g., movement of infected animals)	Many transmission modes, some unknown
Short survival of the agent in the environment	Long survival of the agent in the environment
Fast and inexpensive diagnostic tools and unique clinical signs	Insufficient or expensive diagnostic tools and ambiguous clinical signs
No "healthy" carriers	"Healthy" carriers
High enough morbidity and case-fatality for early detection of the disease	Low morbidity and case fatality
Easy to implement treatment and intervention	No treatment of individuals and no efficient intervention available

Therefore, issues related to people will influence MOSS for zoonoses and for FADs in general.

Economic Considerations

Economic considerations influence all decisions related to MOSSs. All interest groups (government, laboratories, livestock industry or farmer, etc.) involved will consider their costs and benefits regardless of whether this is done by formal economic analysis or by intuition.

Not all groups may be equally interested in all parts of a DCP/DEP, but overall, the economic considerations will include cost-effectiveness of the monitoring, cost-effectiveness of the interventions, short- and long-term costs and benefits, and an awareness of who endures the costs and who gains the benefits.

Although formal economic analysis may not be applied before a DCP/DEP is decided on, it is important to consider the aforementioned issues. If the monitoring and interventions are not cost-effective as well as practical and biologically effective, the DCP/DEP will have minimal chance of success. Furthermore, motivated participants in a DCP/DEP can make the difference between success and failure.

Economic simulation of FMD outbreaks in France has shown that the duration of a ban on the export is a serious cost of epidemics for exporting countries (Mahul and Durand 2000).

Political Issues

Politics may influence decisions about if and when a DCP/DEP is implemented but will rarely influence detailed decisions about the entire MOSS.

The term "politics" is used here in its broadest sense and would include involvement of politicians from federal and local (state/province, county, etc.) governments and of pressure groups (professional and industrial bodies). Media interest often acts as a catalyst for politicians getting involved in decisions about animal health issues like a DCP/DEP.

The involvement of politicians and the media can be increased if the disease is viewed as a human health risk or a food safety issue. Decisions, however, are not exclusively influenced by controlling zoonoses that can trigger interest. If a FAD has an effect on the national economy, politicians may get involved even though there is no threat to human health.

Application of the precautionary principle (Anonymous 2000) is an example of politicians' involvement. The precautionary principle is applied by politicians when faced with an unacceptable risk, scientific uncertainty, and public concerns. In the disease control process, the precautionary principle can be translated as

1. The disease is considered a serious threat to human health.
2. It has major economic effect because the consequences of having the disease are severe.
3. There is scientific uncertainty or limited scientific knowledge.

When the precautionary principle is applied, it may affect the decision about the action taken (do nothing, implement a DCP, or implement a DEP). If action is deemed necessary and a DCP is implemented, the first designed program is unlikely to be the most efficient. Proceeding directly to a DEP may prove very costly if the prevalence is high, the disease spreads rapidly, and there is insufficient knowledge about the effectiveness of the intervention measures. Therefore, the guidelines (Anonymous 2000) to measures based on the precautionary principle include, "Based on an examination of the potential benefits and costs," "Subject to review," and "Assigning responsibility for producing the scientific evidence."

CULTURAL AND SOCIAL FACTORS

Cultural and social factors may have an effect on decisions about MOSSs and, therefore, DCPs/DEPs.

As previously mentioned, MOSSs may be motivated by food safety and quality issues. The consumer's demand for high food-safety documentation and quality might influence the extent of surveillance; for example, there may be markets for *Salmonella*-free chicken in some countries. BSE in cattle is a recent example of how the human health risk has played a key role in the implementation of MOSSs throughout Europe.

Some interventions may be unacceptable to the public in some countries but not in others. For instance,

1. Eradication of wildlife species to eliminate a reservoir: the public in the United Kingdom may not accept the killing of badgers to eradicate TB.
2. Use of depopulation as an alternative to test and slaughter: culling of cattle would not be accepted in India, where cows are sacred.
3. Chemical use, including the use of antibiotics: a consumer issue that may be unacceptable because of concerns about residues in food.

INFRASTRUCTURE

Main Participants

A national or regional MOSS has three main participants: veterinary authorities, laboratories, and livestock industries (including producers). The design of a national MOSS depends on the roles and infrastructure of the three participants.

Veterinary authorities (local, national, or regional) and laboratories (government or private) have unique roles that only they can perform. Legislation and documentation of disease status related to international trade partners rests with the veterinary authorities—more so for OIE list A and B diseases than for production diseases (upper solid/dashed line in Figure 2.3). Diagnostic testing will have to be performed under the guidance of laboratories regardless of the type of disease (lower solid line in Figure 2.3).

MOSSs directly influence the production and market conditions of the livestock industry (farmer organizations, abattoirs, cutting plants, dairies, primary producers, etc.). Therefore, the industry has a keen interest and a key role to perform and, hence, is motivated to influence the design of national MOSSs.

ELEMENTS OF INFRASTRUCTURE

Chapter 3 describes the allocation of administrative and human resources in MOSS. Here there is an assessment of elements of infrastructure (jurisdiction, economic tools, cooperation/competition, expertise [human resources], and demographic/organization) and their potential influence on a MOSS and on compliance and coverage of a DCP/DEP.

The jurisdiction rests with local (region, province, state, etc.), national, or regional authorities. In the simplest case, all legal regulation rests with one authority. This plan may be more complex if more than one authority is involved. But the complexity may be overcome if the legal issues are clearly defined. In the most complex setup, the jurisdiction rests with the authorities; the legal issues are not clearly defined, or are even conflicting (e.g., if regional or national regulations are not implemented locally). If the legal issues are not clearly defined, it may delay implementation of legislation and subsequently influence compliance of a DCP/DEP. That may be the most detrimental factor in the later phase of a DEP when compensation, fines, and penalties are the only means of eliminating the last few cases (Figure 2.4).

Economic incentives (i.e., methods to increase motivation) may influence the timing of when disease is reported and the motivation to comply with the program. The final success of a DEP may depend on a monetary incentive that may be the only means to secure 100% coverage of the population to be exploited and 100% compliance. The tools available to the veterinary authorities and the livestock industries are penalties, fines, and compensation.

Cooperation and competition can be key factors in determining whether a national program is feasible because it has the potential to influence every part of the design (Figure 2.5). Cooperation or competition may influence the design of a DCP/DEP as well as the compliance and coverage of the program. The extremes are full cooperation and strong competition. Full cooperation among the

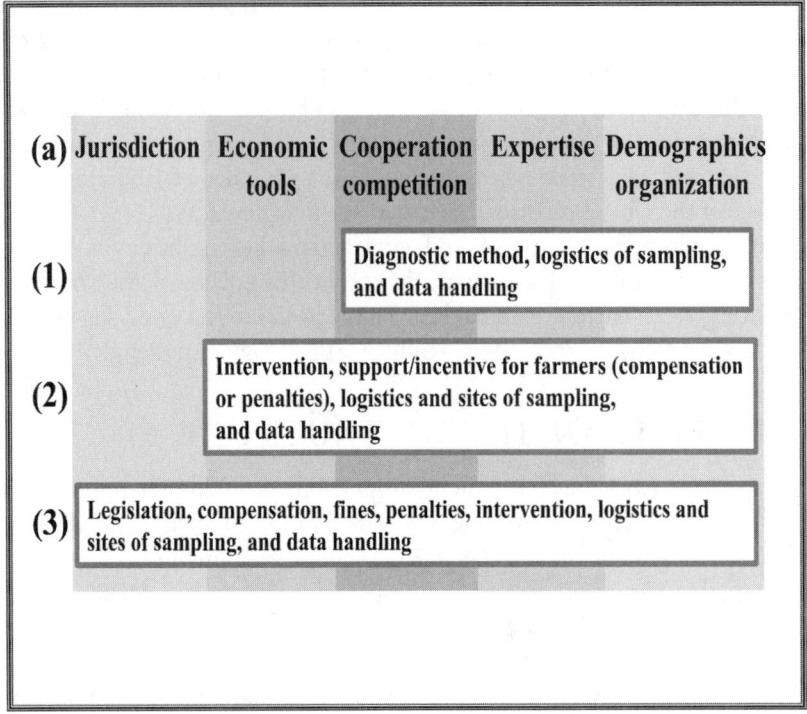

FIGURE 2.4   The step-by-step process of disease control.

main participants and their subgroups tends to promote efficient design of a DCP/DEP with high compliance and coverage. The expertise or human resources needed for the design and maintenance of MOSSs and, thereby, a DCP/DEP may be found with all three main participants, provided sufficient resources are to be found in the country. Where the expertise is found will ideally influence who will do the job rather than how it is done. Some expertise may only be found in academia, and therefore, this source may be applied in design and independent evaluation of a DCP/DEP; not both, however, in the same program.

Demographics and organization may influence how the most efficient monitoring may be designed. Demographics include

- number and organization of veterinarians and veterinary practices, local veterinary organizations, and their reference to authorities
- number of private and state laboratories and their references
- number of animals, farms, abattoirs, dairies, and slaughter market (etc.) and their locations

- and organization of farmers' abattoirs/dairies (e.g., in a cooperative structure).

The demographics vary among countries; therefore, an efficient DCP/DEP in one country may not be applicable in another.

INFORMATION

In the perfect situation, all facts about the disease, population of interest, economics, other issues relating to people, and infrastructure would be known to decision makers so they can make optimal decisions throughout the disease control process. However, we usually only approach that perfect knowledge toward the end of an eradication program or when the time from detection of disease to an implemented DCP is long enough to gain that knowledge.

The precautionary principle mentioned above is applied by politicians to overcome scientific uncertainty. They may decide to start a DCP or DEP although faced with lack of knowledge about the nature of the disease and infrastructure. This lack of knowledge may influence the decision about control strategy, monitoring, and intervention and, thereby, the complete design of the program. Recent examples include BSE in the European Union and *Salmonella* in Denmark. Both diseases were considered a threat to human health at the time when DCPs were implemented. The merit of this approach may be that the risk to human health may be minimized but the downside is that the most efficient DCP/DEP is unlikely to be applied from the start. This can however, be somewhat overcome if new science-based knowledge is constantly sought, published, incorporated, and implemented in the program and if the changes to the program can be communicated to the public.

RATIONALE FOR USING THE DCM

COMMUNICATION METHOD

The rationale for using the disease control model is to communicate issues of the DCP (Figure 2.5). It may help to communicate that FAD control or eradication, for example, is a dynamic process; that changes in control strategy, monitoring, and intervention are a natural part of the process; and that changes can be a reaction to previous success or failure of the program or a reaction to newly acquired knowledge.

As indicated above, the cooperation/competition among the three main participants may influence most parts of the design of a DCP/DEP, the compliance, and the coverage. For a DCP/DEP to be effective and efficient, the

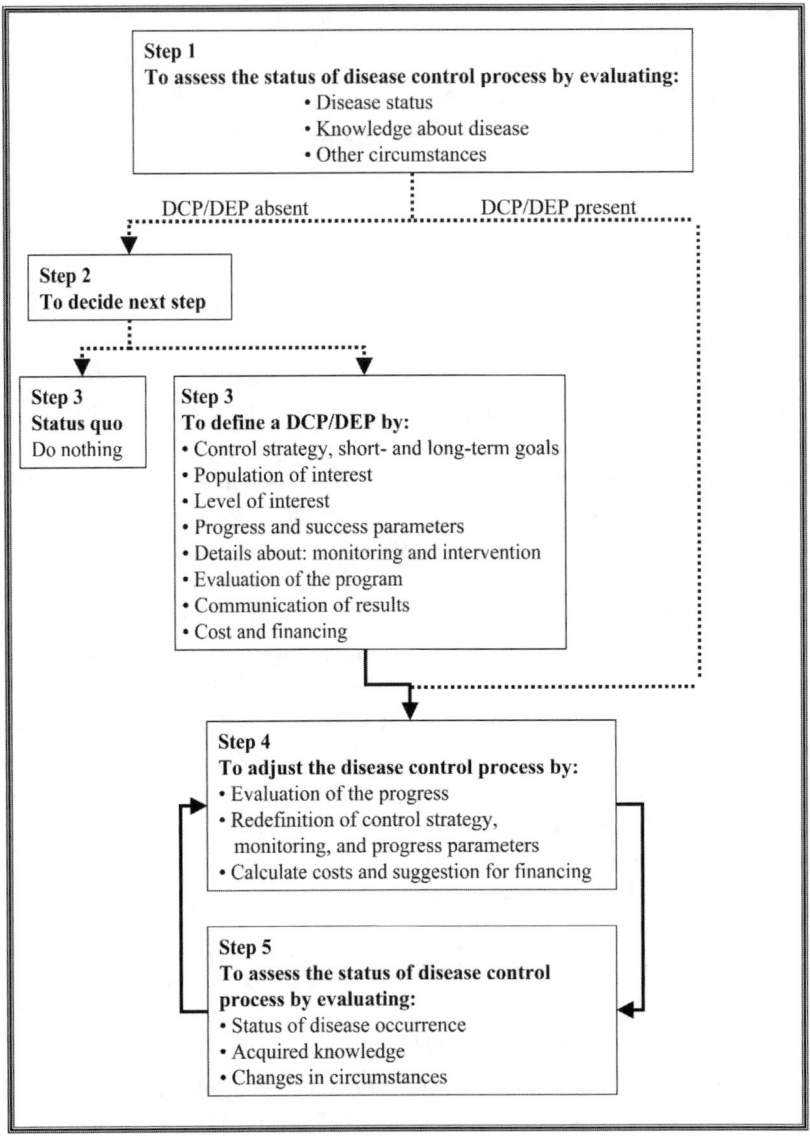

Step 1
To assess the status of disease control process by evaluating:
- Disease status
- Knowledge about disease
- Other circumstances

DCP/DEP absent ⋯⋯⋯⋯⋯⋯⋯⋯⋯⋯ DCP/DEP present ⋯⋯⋯

Step 2
To decide next step

Step 3
Status quo
Do nothing

Step 3
To define a DCP/DEP by:
- Control strategy, short- and long-term goals
- Population of interest
- Level of interest
- Progress and success parameters
- Details about: monitoring and intervention
- Evaluation of the program
- Communication of results
- Cost and financing

Step 4
To adjust the disease control process by:
- Evaluation of the progress
- Redefinition of control strategy,
  monitoring, and progress parameters
- Calculate costs and suggestion for financing

Step 5
To assess the status of disease control
process by evaluating:
- Status of disease occurrence
- Acquired knowledge
- Changes in circumstances

FIGURE 2.5   Five elements of infrastructure that influence the design of monitoring and surveillance and thereby DCP/DEP.

agricultural and veterinary community participants need to be able to communicate quickly and efficiently; therefore, a communication method is relevant. Sometimes, they even have to be able to communicate with the public outside the agricultural world (e.g., doctors, consumers and their organizations, lawyers, and politicians), and again, various forms of communication may be necessary.

CIRCUMSTANCES

Awareness of what circumstances may influence decisions throughout a FAD outbreak in a specific country may be a tool to prepare for the situation by highlighting critical points; for example, deficient knowledge about infrastructure; social or cultural factors that make some interventions impossible; and that for well-known diseases, expertise may be maintained.

Knowledge of the circumstances that influence decisions may be useful in communicating the rationale behind the design of a program to bodies within the country and internationally. Furthermore, it may explain why a program may not be designed in the same way in two otherwise similar countries.

THE DISEASE CONTROL PROCESS: STEP BY STEP

Application of the disease control model and assessment of circumstances would be a method to keep a disease control process dynamic.

For a FAD or emerging disease, the first step would be to assess the status of the disease control process (Figure 2.5) and to apply the disease control model to visualize the status of the disease control process.

In the absence of a DCP/DEP, a decision should be whether to maintain status quo and do nothing or to define a DCP/DEP. In the definition of a DCP/DEP, decisions are made about the need for a standard for capital allocation.

If a DCP/DEP were present, the next step would be to adjust the process, document changes, and communicate the changes (step 4 in Figure 2.5). The adjustment of the process may include evaluation of the progress, achieved parameters, and fulfillment of short- and long-term goals. The step may require redefinition of control strategy and short- and long-term goals. Calculation of expected cost and suggestions for financing the program are part of this step.

The following steps would be iterations of assessment of the disease control process (step 4 in Figure 2.5) and adjustment of the process (step 5 in Figure 2.5).

The disease control process will end when the adjustment in step 4 (Figure 2.5) is completed because disease-free status has been achieved and the control strategy will be the prevention of reintroduction alone or when it is decided that with the present knowledge and under the present circumstances, disease control is not feasible.

BIBLIOGRAPHY

Anonymous. 2000. Commission of the European Communities, 2000. Communication from the Commission on the Precautionary Principle. February 2, 2000, Brussels, 02.02.2000 COM.

Christensen, J. 2001. Epidemiological concepts regarding disease monitoring and surveillance. Acta Vet Scand Suppl. 94:11–16.

Mahul O., Durand B. 2000. Simulated economic consequences of foot-and-mouth disease epidemics and their public control in France. Prev Vet Med 47:23–38.

Martin S.W., Eves J.A., Dolan L.A., Hammond R.F., Griffin J.M., Collins J.D., Shoukri M.M. 1997. The association between the bovine tuberculosis status of herds in the East Offaly Project Area, and the distance to badger setts, 1988–1993. Prev Vet Med 31:113–125.

Paterson B.M., Morris R.S. 1995. Interactions between beef cattle and simulated tuberculous possums on pasture. N Z Vet J. 43:28–29.

Planning Survey, Surveillance, and Monitoring Systems— Roles and Requirements

C. Zepeda and M.D. Salman

INTRODUCTION

Monitoring systems collect, analyze, and disseminate information on animal health related events. Disease surveillance implies the detection of these events and specific actions to address them. Therefore, monitoring systems are an integral part of disease surveillance systems (Doherr and Audigé 2001; Martin et al. 1987; Noordhuizen et al. 1997)

When planning the implementation of monitoring and surveillance systems (MOSSs) several questions need to be asked:

1. Why are disease surveillance and monitoring systems needed?
2. Which diseases should be considered?

Animal Population Health Institute
College of Veterinary Medicine and Biomedical Sciences
Colorado State University

3. What type of data should be collected?
4. Who is going to use the information?
5. What will be the uses of that information?
6. Will the system have national or local coverage?
7. How is the system going to be financed?
8. Is the existing infrastructure adequate?
9. How will the system's efficacy be assessed?
10. What is the legal basis for implementing such a system?

This chapter will attempt to answer these questions and provide a guide for the planning and implementation of disease surveillance and monitoring systems that will be efficient and that will provide credible information for decision making.

NEED FOR ANIMAL DISEASE SURVEILLANCE AND MONITORING

Animal disease surveillance and monitoring have been essential activities for official veterinary services. However, in recent years, increased trade in animals and animal products has increased the importance of international disease reporting.

The information that the system generates must increase the understanding of the occurrence of disease and be used to improve animal health through appropriate actions. In other words, disease surveillance is the tool that provides information for planning disease control and eradication programs.

The World Trade Organization's (WTO) Agreement on the Application of Sanitary and Phytosanitary Measures (SPS Agreement) has changed the way animal health requirements for international trade in animals and animal products are applied internationally. The SPS Agreement introduced several important concepts such as regionalization, risk analysis, harmonization, equivalence, and transparency that affect the organization and infrastructure of veterinary services worldwide (WTO 1995). Of these, regionalization and risk analysis are the most significant, as both have an immediate relationship with veterinary epidemiology and, more directly, with disease surveillance systems.

The SPS Agreement recognizes the Office International des Epizooties (OIE) as the international organization responsible for drafting international animal health standards. The SPS agreement requires that animal health decisions are science based. This has placed disease surveillance systems, and veterinary epidemiology in general, at the core of animal health–related decisions (Zepeda et al. 2001). Today, efficient disease surveillance and monitoring systems are the basis for trust in international trade in animals and animal products.

In 1924, the OIE was established by an international agreement signed by 28 countries; by 2001, membership had risen to 158 member countries. The OIE's main objectives have been to

- guarantee the transparency of animal disease status worldwide by informing governments of the occurrence and course of animal diseases throughout the world and of ways to control these diseases;
- collect, analyze, and disseminate veterinary scientific information;
- promote and coordinate research in surveillance and control of animal diseases throughout the world—this task is undertaken by specialist commissions and working groups, with support from collaborating centers and reference laboratories, as well as by the organization of meetings of experts and the publication of scientific articles;
- guarantee the sanitary safety of world trade by developing sanitary rules for international trade in animals and animal products (OIE 2001b).

More recently, the OIE has received the mandate to develop standards for food safety and animal welfare.

All OIE member countries have the obligation to report the occurrence of all list A and B diseases (Appendix 3.1). List A diseases are defined as transmissible diseases that have the potential for very serious and rapid spread, irrespective of national borders; that are of serious socioeconomic or public health consequence; and that are of major importance in the international trade of animals and animal products. List B diseases are defined as transmissible diseases that are considered to be of socioeconomic or public health importance within countries and that are significant in the international trade of animals and animal products (OIE 2001a).

There are three different types of reports (OIE 2001c).

1. **Emergency reports:** Countries must notify the OIE Central Bureau within 24 hours of the occurrence of a significant epidemiological event. Thereafter, they must provide progress reports on a weekly basis until such time as the situation becomes stable or the disease concerned has been eradicated. The sending of weekly reports should stop once a disease has become enzootic. The form can also be used to report the lifting of sanitary measures when it is considered that all the recorded outbreaks have been eliminated. The central bureau immediately sends a summary of the warning message by e-mail to member countries. In addition, the OIE publishes a weekly disease information leaflet that is sent to all member countries and is also available online.
2. **Monthly reports:** Countries need to provide information on the absence or presence of list A diseases and, where appropriate, a compilation of

data relating to diseases not on this list that have been the subject of emergency or follow-up reports during the month in question. For list A diseases that are enzootic, no emergency or follow-up reports should be sent.

3. **Yearly report:** Once a year, member countries submit a written report summarizing the most important information on their disease control efforts as well as a complete report on the occurrence of list A and B diseases in their territories.

It is obvious that international disease reporting, although extremely important, is not the only goal for a MOSS. Surveillance systems provide valuable information for country decision-making and for monitoring progress in control and eradication of economically important diseases.

CRITERIA FOR INCLUSION OF DISEASES FOR SURVEILLANCE

Realistically, not all diseases can be the object of surveillance and monitoring. Although all OIE member countries have the obligation to report on the occurrence of list A and B diseases, only a few of these are usually under active or passive surveillance systems. Priorities and criteria for the inclusion of diseases for surveillance and monitoring vary from country to country and between different regions of the world.

In general, the criteria for the inclusion of diseases in surveillance systems have been based on their potential to have a public health effect (e.g., zoonotic diseases), diseases that significantly affect production, and diseases that limit international trade. It is the role of the official veterinary service along with producers' groups and public health officials to establish priorities and balance the need to obtain disease information with budget limitations.

The type of data that the MOSS will collect and the uses of the information need to be clearly defined in the design phase before implementation. Different users usually will expect different outputs from the system. An ideal MOSS should gather data on the agent, the host, and the environment (Hueston 1993). Data collected should at least include the number of cases, species, population at risk, type of production system, location of cases, laboratory confirmation, and type of test used.

A MOSS with national coverage may have different emphasis in certain regions of the country based on the progress of the disease control and eradication programs. Thus, in an endemic area, the system may rely more on passive reporting of cases, whereas in areas approaching eradication and in disease-free areas, greater emphasis will be placed on active surveillance through the use of statistically based surveys.

LEGAL BASIS

A MOSS must have a legal framework to support it. Different countries may have different legal systems, but in general, the "Animal Health Law" provides the broad framework for the operation of the veterinary service, including disease monitoring and surveillance.

A more detailed regulation stemming from the broad legal framework must describe the activities to be performed by the MOSS. This regulation should include a list of notifiable diseases. The composition of this list may vary between countries. Ideally, notifiable diseases should include diseases that are exotic to the country, diseases under official control or eradication programs, and diseases considered important for monitoring purposes.

FUNDING

Traditionally, disease monitoring and surveillance systems have been considered the core of the veterinary services "intelligence" and, therefore, an activity that is not susceptible to privatization. Although the primary responsibility for disease monitoring and surveillance lies with the official veterinary service, private sector participation is essential in ensuring a rapid response. Funding for targeted surveillance can and should be shared by the interested industries. In the developing world, funding for surveillance activities is often hard to obtain. It is evident that the official sector cannot totally finance the activities necessary to establish a credible disease monitoring and surveillance system. Some alternatives that are currently being used are

- accreditation of private professionals to carry out official actions such as sample collection for various diseases or testing for tuberculosis;
- privatization of services under the regulation and supervision of the state, including diagnostic laboratories to support official eradication efforts;
- and schemes of mixed financial participation with specific objectives such as disease eradication campaigns (Zepeda 1998).

Many of the disease surveillance activities can be performed under a scheme with private sector participation. In many countries, particularly where intensive production systems and subsistence farming co-exist, there is still a need for direct official participation at all levels of the MOSS. This is not to say that private funding cannot be obtained to perform these activities.

Intensive production farmers have a direct interest in helping control disease at the subsistence farming level as much as in their own establishments.

Access to export markets is the most important incentive for private sector participation. When an importing country assesses the sanitary status of an exporting country or zone, great emphasis is placed on the efficacy of the surveillance system in detecting the reintroduction of disease. The MOSS must be able to demonstrate the absence of disease at both the subsistence and intensive production systems. Disease freedom claims must be based on a combination of active and passive collection of the required data and information for the surveillance system. Surveys to support disease freedom claims need to cover both types of production systems; therefore, it is in the intensive farmers' best interest to fund active surveillance in subsistence production systems

Small-scale producers often will not be able to access export markets; their incentive for reporting is the increased production and reduced mortality achieved by the control or eradication of disease.

UNDERREPORTING

Underreporting is the single most important constraint to a MOSS. Mistrust and lack of knowledge are the roots of underreporting. Producer education is central in promoting disease reporting: What should be notified? Where to? What happens if disease is detected on my premises?

Lack of appropriate compensation also leads to underreporting. Veterinary services often do not have the funds to compensate producers for the loss of animals that need to be destroyed to contain an outbreak, let alone to compensate for the loss of production and time needed to get back to full production. Sadly, on many occasions previous experience leading to the application of drastic measures to eliminate disease outbreaks is the main reason for not reporting disease.

Obviously, funding is the most important element in developing trust. In some countries government funds cover for direct losses resulting from the destruction of animals, and farmer organizations or insurance cover the loss of production. Unfortunately, in most developing countries, even the funding to cover stamping-out policies is not available.

TRAINING

The basis for success in any MOSS is a well-qualified force operating at all levels of the system. Training can be targeted for different audiences: decision-makers, epidemiologists, field veterinarians, and laboratory personnel.

Decision-makers must be able to understand the importance of setting a MOSS, the diseases that should be under the system, and the elements needed to interpret and apply the information generated by the system.

Epidemiologists must be knowledgeable on survey design, interpretation of diagnostic tests—and of diagnostic test sensitivity and specificity in particular, predictive values, and herd sensitivity and specificity as well as the general epidemiology of diseases under the MOSS.

Field personnel need to understand the importance of surveys as a tool to demonstrate the disease status of a country or zone. In this respect, gathering information on population data is extremely important. Often the lack of denominator data is one of the most significant constraints to appropriate survey design. Field personnel must also gather information on general terms of animal movements into and out of the zone under the MOSS. Another essential task at this level of the system is to raise producers' awareness of the importance of disease notification and the procedures to follow if a disease is suspected.

A well-qualified laboratory is essential to any MOSS. Laboratory personnel need to be knowledgeable in the different diagnostic procedures for all diseases covered by the system. The laboratory needs to understand the limitations and applicability of diagnostic tests and to help the epidemiologists in interpreting laboratory results.

COMMUNICATION

Analysis transforms data into information. It is said that information is power; this is true, but only if the information flows from the sources to the users and vice versa. The mere accumulation of information with no useful output is useless and will erode the trust placed on the MOSS system. Routine periodic information in the form of regular (weekly, monthly, or yearly) reports to all users of the system will improve the acceptability, representativeness, data quality, and usefulness of the system—important elements in the evaluation of MOSS systems (Centers for Disease Control and Prevention [CDC] 2001; Thacker et al. 1988)

ASSESSMENT OF MOSS

Periodic evaluations of the system will provide information to recognize and address situations that hinder its efficiency and efficacy. The CDC recently published guidelines for the evaluation of public health MOSS systems (CDC 2001). The CDC lists several criteria to assess the performance of the system. Table 3.1 summarizes these criteria.

Additional elements for assessment of animal health–related MOSS systems have been proposed (Hueston 1993). These are based on factors related to agent surveillance, host monitoring, environmental assessment, and the epidemiological delivery system.

TABLE 3.1   Criteria for Assessing the Performance of Monitoring and Surveillance Systems

Criteria	Description
Usefulness	Description of the system's contribution to the prevention and control of diseases
Simplicity	Structure and ease of operation. Surveillance systems should be as simple as possible while still meeting their objectives.
Flexibility	Ability to adapt to changing information needs or operating conditions with little additional time, personnel, or allocated funds.
Data quality	Refers to the completeness and validity of the data recorded in the surveillance system.
Acceptability	Reflects the willingness of persons and organizations to participate in the surveillance system.
Sensitivity	Refers to the proportion of cases of a disease (or other health-related event) detected by the surveillance system. Alternatively, sensitivity can refer to the ability to detect outbreaks, including the ability to monitor changes in the number of cases over time
Predictive value positive	Refers to proportion of reported cases that actually have the health-related event under surveillance (i.e. that match the case definition).
Representativeness	Ability to describe the occurrence of a health-related event over time and its distribution in the population by place and species.
Timeliness	Reflects the speed between steps in a surveillance system.
Stability	Refers to the reliability (i.e., the ability to collect, manage, and provide data properly without failure) and availability (the ability to be operational when it is needed) of the surveillance system.

Note. Adapted from Centers for Disease Control and Prevention 2001 and Thacker et al. 1988.

In addition, the MOSS needs to generate information useful for animal health risk analysis for import–export decisions.

CONCLUSIONS

Monitoring and surveillance systems are the spinal cord of a veterinary service and an indispensable tool for the control and eradication of diseases. More recently, MOSSs have gained increased importance as the single most important element in transparency for certification for export of animals and animal products. The SPS Agreement requires that all member countries notify the

OIE of changes in their animal health status. Transparency in the detection and reporting of disease generates trust among trading countries. Trust is, and should remain, the basis for credibility in the certification process.

BIBLIOGRAPHY

Centers for Disease Control and Prevention. 2001. Updated guidelines for evaluating public health surveillance systems. Centers for Disease Control and Prevention; http://www.cdc.gov/mmwr/preview/mmwrhtml/rr5013a1.htm.

Doherr M.G., Audigé L. 2001. Monitoring and surveillance for rare health-related events: A review from the veterinary perspective. Phil Trans R Soc Lond B Biol Sci 356:1097–1106.

Hueston W.D. 1993. Assessment of national systems for the surveillance and monitoring of animal health. Rev Sci Technol 12(4):1187–1196.

Martin S.W., Meek A.H., Willeberg P. 1987. Veterinary Epidemiology. Iowa State University Press, Ames.

Noordhuizen J.P.T.M., Frankena K., van der Hoofd C.M., Graat E.A.M. 1997. Application of quantitative methods in veterinary epidemiology. Wageningen Press, Wageningen, The Netherlands.

Office International des Epizooties. 2001a. International Animal Health Code. Office International des Epizooties, Paris; http://www.oie.int.

Office International des Epizooties. 2001b. OIE at a glance. Office International des Epizooties, Paris; http://www.oie.int.

Office International des Epizooties. 2001c. Manual for animal disease reporting to the OIE. Office International des Epizooties, Paris; http://www.oie.int.

Thacker S.B., Parrish R.G., Trowbridge F.L. 1988. A method for evaluating systems of epidemiological surveillance. World Health Stat Q 41:11–18.

World Trade Organization. 1995. Agreement on the Application of Sanitary and Phytosanitary Measures. World Trade Organization; http://www.wto.org.

Zepeda C. 1998. Perspectives of veterinary services in Latin America in the face of globalization. Second FAO Electronic Conference on Veterinary Services; http://www.fao.org/WAICENT/FAOINFO/AGRICULT/AGA/AGAH/Vets-l-2/Contents.htm.

Zepeda C., Salman M., Ruppanner R. 2001 International trade, animal health and veterinary epidemiology: Challenges and opportunities. Prev Vet Med 48:261–271.

APPENDIX 3.1

Office International des Epizooties Classification of Reportable Diseases

List and disease

List A

- Foot and mouth disease
- Swine vesicular disease
- Peste des petits ruminants
- Lumpy skin disease
- Bluetongue
- African horse sickness
- Classical swine fever
- Newcastle disease
- Vesicular stomatitis
- Rinderpest
- Contagious bovine pleuropneumonia
- Rift Valley fever
- Sheep pox and goat pox
- African swine fever
- Highly pathogenic avian influenza

List B

Multiple species diseases
- Anthrax
- Aujeszky s disease
- Echinococcosis/hydatidosis
- Heartwater
- Leptospirosis
- New world screwworm (*Cochliomyia hominivorax*)
- Old world screwworm (*Chrysomya bezziana*)
- Paratuberculosis
- Q fever
- Rabies
- Trichinellosis

Cattle diseases
- Bovine anaplasmosis
- Bovine babesiosis
- Bovine brucellosis
- Bovine cysticercosis
- Bovine genital campylobacteriosis
- Bovine spongiform encephalopathy
- Bovine tuberculosis
- Dermatophilosis
- Enzootic bovine leukosis
- Haemorrhagic septicaemia
- Infectious bovine rhinotracheitis/ infectious pustular vulvovaginitis
- Malignant catarrhal fever
- Theileriosis
- Trichomonosis
- Trypanosomosis (tsetse-borne)

Sheep and goat diseases
- Caprine and ovine brucellosis (excluding *Brucella ovis*)
- Caprine arthritis/encephalitis
- Contagious agalactia
- Contagious caprine pleuropneumonia
- Enzootic abortion of ewes (ovine chlamydiosis)
- Maedi-visna
- Nairobi sheep disease

Equine diseases
- Contagious equine metritis
- Dourine
- Epizootic lymphangitis
- Equine encephalomyelitis (Eastern and Western)
- Equine infectious anaemia
- Equine influenza
- Equine piroplasmosis
- Equine rhinopneumonitis

List and disease

Sheep and goat diseases (contd.)
- Ovine epididymitis (*Brucella ovis*)
- Ovine pulmonary adenomatosis
- Salmonellosis (*Salmonella abortusovis*)
- Scrapie

Swine diseases
- Atrophic rhinitis of swine
- Enterovirus encephalomyelitis
- Porcine brucellosis
- Porcine cysticercosis
- Porcine reproductive and respiratory syndrome
- Transmissible gastroenteritis

Lagomorph diseases
- Myxomatosis
- Rabbit haemorrhagic disease
- Tularemia

Fish diseases
- Epizootic haematopoietic necrosis
- Infectious haematopoietic necrosis
- *Oncorhynchus masou* virus disease
- Spring viraemia of carp
- Viral haemorrhagic septicaemia

Equine diseases (contd.)
- Equine viral arteritis
- Glanders
- Horse mange
- Horse pox
- Japanese encephalitis
- Surra (*Trypanosoma evansi*)
- Venezuelan equine encephalomyelitis

Avian diseases
- Avian chlamydiosis
- Avian infectious bronchitis
- Avian infectious laryngotracheitis
- Avian mycoplasmosis (*Mycoplasma gallisepticum*)
- Avian tuberculosis
- Duck virus enteritis
- Duck virus hepatitis
- Fowl cholera
- Fowl pox
- Fowl typhoid
- Infectious bursal disease (Gumboro disease)
- Marek's disease
- Pullorum disease

Bee diseases
- Acariosis of bees
- American foulbrood
- European foulbrood
- Nosemosis of bees
- Varroosis

Mollusk diseases
- Bonamiosis (*Bonamia ostreae, B. exitiosus, Mikrocytos roughleyi*)
- Marteiliosis (*Marteilia refringens, M. sydneyi*)
- Mikrocytosis (*Mikrocytos mackini*)
- MSX disease (*Haplosporidium nelsoni*)
- Perkinsosis (*Perkinsus marinus, P. olseni/atlanticus*)

(Appendix 3.1 continued)

List and disease

Crustacean diseases
- Taura syndrome
- White spot disease
- Yellowhead disease

Other diseases
- Leishmaniosis

Note. From Office International des Epizooties 2001c.

Sampling Considerations in Surveys and Monitoring and Surveillance Systems

A. Cameron,[1] I. Gardner,[2] M.G. Doherr,[3] and B. Wagner[4]

SAMPLING METHODS AND SAMPLE SIZE

This chapter deals with sampling, or the process of selecting a number of elements from a group (e.g., animals) for a survey or a monitoring and surveillance system (MOSS). First, a number of important concepts are introduced. This introduction is followed by a discussion of different practical techniques for selecting a sample. The third part discusses sampling in relation to a number of different survey designs, with special reference to the question of sample size. Finally, we examine a number of special situations that require different sampling approaches.

[1]Ausvet Animal Health Services, Wentworth Falls, New South Wales 2782, Australia
[2]Department of Medicine and Epidemiology, School of Veterinary Medicine, University of California, Davis, CA 95616
[3]Department of Veterinary Clinical Medicine, University of Bern, Bern, Switzerland CH-3001
[4]USDA:APHIS:VS:CEAH, Mail Stop #2E7, 2150 Centre Avenue, Building B, Fort Collins, CO 80526–8117

Sampling Concepts

Populations

For the purpose of this section, a population may be broadly defined as a group of elements that share some common defined characteristic. To usefully apply the idea of a population, it must be finite in size and clearly defined in space and time, such that for every element in the universe, we may determine whether it is a member of the population or not.

This definition usually includes components of what, where, and when (although the latter may be implicit).

Note that under this broad definition, a population does not have to be homogeneous, nor even consist of tangible objects. A few examples will serve to illustrate different population definitions:

- **All the cattle in the United Kingdom:** This identifies what (all cattle), where (in the United Kingdom), and implies when (at the notional time point when a particular study was carried out).
- **Foot and mouth disease (FMD)–susceptible species in sub-Saharan Africa:** Note that this is not a homogenous population with regards to species—cattle, sheep, pigs, and a range of wild ruminants are all included.
- **Chickens in a particular cage on a specified intensive layer farm:** The size of this population is likely to be small—only two or three chickens—however, it is still a valid definition of a population.
- **Farm visits made by government veterinary staff in Australia during 2000:** This population is made up of events, not animals, people, or farms. This population definition is valid, as long as it is supported by appropriate definitions of what constitutes a farm and what is meant by government veterinary staff.
- **Consignments of buffalo transported from Vietnam to Thailand in December 2001:** This definition identifies groups of animals involved in events (animal transport).
- **All the fish in the ocean:** A large, uncountable, yet finite population (as long as we have a clear idea of what we mean by fish, whether seas are included, and where we delineate the lines between river, estuary, and ocean).
- **All swine herds in Denmark on January 1, 2002:** Herds are an appropriate population if the individual animal is not of interest and if all interventions will be at the herd level.

In a MOSS, it is often useful to define a number of related populations.

Target Population (Or Population of Interest)
This is the population about which we are asking questions and ultimately making inferences. Usually, it is the same as the population at risk of being af-

fected by the condition being studied, but it also can be a high-risk subgroup within a larger population.

Study Population
This is the population that is actually studied. In a survey, this is the population from which a sample is drawn.

Ideally, the study population is the same as the target population, but often this is not the case. For example, a target population may be all the FMD-susceptible animals in an area. For practical reasons, it may not be possible to identify and capture wild animals (e.g., deer or wild boar) or even include small-holder domestic animals (e.g., pet sheep, cattle, or pigs) in the study. The study population would therefore only include FMD-susceptible commercially farmed animals in the area.

The difference between the target and study population is important for the interpretation of results of a survey or MOSS. For example, a well-designed survey may be able to draw valid conclusions about the study population, but these conclusions cannot be automatically extended to the target population if the two populations are substantially different.

Census Versus Sampling

Once the target and study populations have been identified, it is necessary to gather data about that population. One approach is to collect information from every single member of the study population—a process known as taking a census. Apart from collecting complete information about a population, the advantage of a census is that there is no uncertainty associated with the results caused by sampling error (although other sources of uncertainty such as measurement error, nonresponse, or data management errors may still exist). If a study of a population of 10,000 horses found that 345 truly had a particular disease, then the observed prevalence was exactly 3.45%. The prevalence is known precisely and not open to doubt, and there is no need for complicated statistics to make estimates about the population. The main disadvantage of conducting a census is that, except in very small populations, they are slow and very expensive. In all but a few cases, gathering census data usually is not cost effective, as data of the required quality can be collected much more cheaply using a sample.

A sample is defined as a group of elements selected from the study population. Data are collected only from the sample. The key advantage of sampling is that information about a population can be gathered much more quickly and cheaply than by using a census. If the sample is selected correctly, the information from the sample can be used to reliably estimate characteristics of the population. The disadvantage of using a sample is that the characteristics of the population are not known for certain. In our example above with a population of 10,000 horses, if a sample of 100 were taken and three horses were identified as truly diseased, we could make two conclusions: that 3% of the sample was diseased (i.e., a prevalence of 3%), and that about 3% of the population is likely to diseased.

There is no doubt about the first conclusion, as it is a statement of fact. The second is open to some debate. Much of the rest of this section on sampling is devoted to clarifying what the word *about* actually means.

Sample Census

Population studies sometimes employ a technique confusingly described as a sample census. Such studies in fact use samples (although often large ones) but are interested in collecting the type of information normally collected by censuses.

Census-based Surveillance Systems

Some MOSSs are based on the principle of collecting complete information. Mandatory disease notification systems, disease registries, and examination of animals at slaughter are examples of these. These systems are based on the assumption that every member of the population is under observation, and when an animal becomes affected with a specific disease, a report is made. Given that the units in the population can be described, the data may therefore be thought of as census data, and measures of prevalence or incidence are not subject to uncertainty attributable to sampling. Unfortunately, it is rare that all disease events in a population are captured by such systems, and sometimes the size of the population (e.g., number of herds) is not truly known. This means that what might be interpreted as a census is often a sample. The case ascertainment rate (the proportion of all cases that are identified by the surveillance system) is used to adjust the results, but some bias and uncertainty are introduced because the sample may not be truly representative of the population.

Clustering and Subpopulations

Because of a range of biological, environmental, economic, and management factors, animal populations are clustered in groups. Furthermore, this clustering may occur at several levels. For instance, the pig population of Europe is largely clustered into a number of highly intensive pig production regions. Within these regions the population is divided into farms, each of which may have animals housed in a number of sheds. Animals in sheds may be further grouped into pens. Moreover, some farms have multiple production sites, which introduce an additional level of hierarchy. Animals within clusters have a disease risk that is more likely to be similar than the disease risk for animals in different clusters.

When developing a MOSS, it is therefore necessary to take disease clustering into account. A system that aims to measure the animal-level prevalence of disease may not provide useful information if it does not consider farm-level clustering. For instance, many infectious diseases cluster at a farm level. The animal-level prevalence in affected farms may be relatively high, but only a small proportion of farms are affected, whereas most farms have a prevalence of zero. To better describe this situation, it is necessary to measure both the farm-level prevalence (proportion of farms with animals affected by the disease) and the animal-level prevalence within farms (or the within-farm prevalence).

For example, instead of considering the total pig population, we consider first the population of pig farms and then the population of pigs within each farm. The process can be extended to smaller groups of animals and is the basis for multistage sampling techniques, which are described in subsequent sections.

Because of clustering of the population, different approaches might be necessary if the objective of a survey is to estimate prevalence at all levels. However, a survey often might only focus on estimation of prevalence at the farm level because of extreme clustering and because intervention will be at the farm rather than the individual level.

Bias and Precision

When a sample is used to gather information about a population, the result is always subject to uncertainty because of the sampling process. If a sample is selected, the animals examined, and disease prevalence within the sample calculated, it can be used to estimate the prevalence in the population. However, if another sample is drawn from the same population, we are likely to get a different answer because different animals were examined. This process could be continued, and each time a sample is drawn, a slightly different result would be obtained. The range of different results is the cause of the uncertainty and the reason why we can only estimate population prevalence from a sample. In this case, it is important to have some way of measuring how good our estimate is. The quality of an estimate is expressed using two measures: bias and precision.

If a population were repeatedly sampled using a particular sampling approach and an estimate of the prevalence calculated for each sample, a range of different estimates would be produced. The mean of these estimates can then be calculated. If a good sampling technique is used, the mean of the repeated estimates is very close to the true value (which can only be determined by using a census). With a poor sampling technique, the mean of the estimates is distinctly different from the true population value. The difference between the mean of repeated estimates and the true value is termed "bias," and a good sampling technique is one that is unbiased. A number of other sources of bias exist, such as measurement error, but poor sampling technique is the most important and often the most avoidable cause of bias. The effect of bias is to over- or underestimate the parameter of interest; for example, prevalence. If decision makers make certain decisions because they assume that the data are correct, the process of disease control can be hindered and unnecessary costs incurred. The problem with sampling bias is that it can usually only be measured by repeatedly sampling the population as well as doing a census to find the true population value. In reality, a census will rarely be done, so inferences about the likelihood of a sampling bias mostly will be based on a consideration of whether the sample was sufficiently representative of the population.

One goal to remember when designing a sampling technique should, therefore, always be to avoid bias. The only way to avoid bias is to ensure that the sample is representative of the population. Representativeness means that the characteristics of the sample are similar to those of the population. For instance, a sample that is representative of the population with respect to gender would have the genders in the same proportion as in the population. If the genders are in the same proportion, the sample still may not be representative with respect to age (the population and sample have different age distributions). If both age and gender are similarly distributed, there are many other characteristics (weight, breed, production, management, genetics, etc.) that may or may not be similarly distributed. Ensuring similar distributions of these and of the many other possible characteristics requires prior knowledge of the distribution of the characteristic in the population. However, from the point of view of the study, only one characteristic is relevant: that characteristic being studied (e.g., disease or antibody status). If the distribution of the characteristic of interest is the same in the study population and the sample, the study will not be biased. Unfortunately, it is not possible to guarantee that the sample is representative with respect to the characteristic of interest without first doing a census, making any subsequent sampling irrelevant.

Precision

Precision is a measure of how variable the estimates from repeated samples are. Although we can expect the estimates from different samples to vary, if most of them are very close to each other, we have a precise estimate, and we can be highly confident that (in the absence of bias) estimated values are close to the real value. If, however, the spread of repeated estimates is wide, our estimate is imprecise, and we have less confidence that a particular estimate is close to the real value. Unlike bias, we can measure the precision of our sample without doing a census.

Precision is usually expressed in terms of a 95% confidence interval. If a sample is repeated many times, and a 95% confidence interval is calculated for each estimate, the true value would fall within the calculated confidence intervals 95% of the time. (This is subtly different from the common but incorrect interpretation that we are 95% confident that the true value lies within the interval.)

Clearly, a study with high precision is desirable. However if an estimate has lower precision, it may still be useful, as long as the precision is actually known and can be taken into account when making decisions based on the results. The main factor that controls precision is the sample size, as described in a subsequent section.

Inference

In sampling, inference is the process of assuming that the characteristics observed in a group (or sample) are similar to those in the population from which they were selected. Inference is only valid if the sample is representative of the population. There are two approaches to inference: logical and statistical. Logical inference involves putting forward soundly based arguments as to why the sample may be considered to be similar to, and representative of, the population. Clearly these arguments should include a consideration of reasons why the sample also may not be representative. Logical inference may be used to attempt to infer that characteristics observed in a study population are the same as in a larger target population. Unfortunately, the factors causing some elements of the target population to be excluded from the study population may also mean that the characteristic being studied is different in these elements, resulting in bias.

Statistical inference uses probability theory to determine just how likely it is that the characteristics observed in a sample are similar to those of the source population. Statistical inference can only validly be applied to results for certain sampling designs, as discussed in the section on sampling techniques.

Because most surveys and MOSSs use diagnostic tests, it is important that the effects of test accuracy on inferences be considered in the planning phase. This consideration is especially important if the investigator has multiple tests from which to choose or if the goal is to verify disease freedom. For instance, a test with a sensitivity of 99% and specificity of 99.8% would usually be considered a very accurate test. However if it were used as the basis of a survey to demonstrate that a country was free from disease, and 10,000 animals were tested, you would expect the test to give about 20 positive results, even if the population were completely free from disease. In a prevalence survey, where there is a mixture of truly positive and truly negative animals, most tests will produce both false-positive and false-negative results. Methods to adjust survey data for imperfect sensitivity and specificity are described in a subsequent chapter.

A secondary consideration is the nature of the characteristic being measured. Most tests are concerned with identifying disease or infection, but this is usually done indirectly—based, for example, on clinical signs; hematologic, biochemical, histologic, or immunologic changes; or the detection of pathogens. When a range of different indicators of disease is available, the duration of the change in the diseased state is an important consideration.

For example, a sentinel system is being established to detect the incursion of arboviral diseases; in particular, bluetongue. Two tests are considered: viral isolation and serology. In bluetongue, virus is detectable in the blood for a variable period, but in most animals it is less than 2 weeks. However, antibodies induced by the infection last for many years. If animals were to be tested every 2 months, it would be very easy to fail to detect acute infection, and hence, isolate virus. However, seroconversion would be much easier to detect.

A final consideration is whether the test will be used for herd-level diagnosis or estimation of within-herd prevalence. In the former case, targeted (purposive) sampling of high-risk groups might be appropriate, whereas random sampling will be necessary to estimate within-herd prevalence. Concepts of herd-level sensitivity and specificity and their effects on herd-level diagnosis of disease are described elsewhere (Christensen and Gardner 2000; Martin et al. 1992).

SAMPLING TECHNIQUES

There are many ways in which a sample can be drawn from a population, and these can be conveniently categorized into probability and nonprobability sampling techniques.

Nonprobability

In nonprobability sampling techniques, the choice of which animals (or other elements) to include in a sample is made by the person doing the sampling, based on the specific approach used. There are three commonly used nonprobability sampling approaches.

In **convenience sampling**, the animals that are most convenient are selected for the sample. For example, a survey of lameness in dairy cattle may require sampling of animals. A convenience sample might include the first 10 animals in a herd to enter the milking shed. This is a simple approach, as it is not necessary to wait for the entire herd to pass through the shed. However, such a sample would be severely biased, as the most severely lame animals would be amongst the last to enter the shed.

Purposive sampling involves the selection of animals to meet some determined purpose. For example, to determine the prevalence of ovine paratuberculosis infection in a flock, a sample of sheep with signs of diarrhea ("high-risk" animals) might be selected, as these are judged more likely to be positive on serologic tests or fecal culture. Although this approach might be appropriate if trying to determine whether the infection is present or not, the sample results are likely to overestimate the true within-herd prevalence.

The third nonprobability sampling technique, **haphazard sampling**, is perhaps the most commonly used. It involves the selection of animals haphazardly, or with no apparent plan or reason. This is usually done in the belief that it mimics probability sampling, but is often just as subject to bias as the previous two approaches. This is because, even when attempting not to, the human mind always has a reason for picking an element. Large, difficult-to-handle animals may be subconsciously avoided; farms that are remote or owned by uncooperative farmers may also be excluded. In contrast to convenience samples, which tend to be spatially clustered, haphazard samples tend to be uniformly or evenly distributed, which may introduce new biases.

Nonprobability sampling techniques generally have the appeal of simplicity, but their main disadvantage is that they are unable to reliably generate a truly representative sample. Because of their simplicity, it is sometimes contended that they are less expensive than probability sampling techniques. However, the proportion of survey costs that is attributable to sampling is usually relatively small compared to that of fieldwork and specimen processing. A slight savings in sampling often has little effect on the overall survey cost. More important is the issue of the value of data quality. Although it is very difficult to quantify, it is clear that biased data have a much lower value than representative data; indeed, biased data may be worse than no data if they lead to incorrect inference and poor decision making.

Probability

Probability sampling is formally defined as a sampling scheme in which each member of the study population has a known, nonzero probability of being selected in the sample. In the specific example of simple random sampling, each member of the population has the same probability of being chosen in the sample. To implement this unpredictability, a random selection process is required that takes the decision of which animals to select out of the hands of the person doing the sampling and makes it purely a matter of chance.

Probability sampling has two important advantages. First, it is the only way to reliably select a representative sample from a population (other than by previously testing the entire population). A particular random sample may not always be a good representation of the population, but it gives the best chance of obtaining one and is the only way to avoid sampling bias.

Second, if probability sampling is used, it allows us to appropriately interpret the results of that sample. Every common formula used to analyze data from samples, from the simple estimate of a proportion or mean to complex confidence interval calculations, is based on the assumption that the data have been collected using probability sampling. Similarly, the process of statistical inference from the sample to the population is only valid if probability sampling has been used.

Random Sampling Techniques

Simple random sampling is the technique from which all other probability sampling techniques are derived. The two requirements are a sampling frame and a method of randomization.

A sampling frame is a list of all elements in the study population and is usually numbered sequentially to assist selection (although the numbering may be only conceptual). Characteristics of a good sampling frame are that it has no omissions (the entire population is listed), that it has no duplications (each element is listed once only), and that each element is uniquely identified.

Many sampling frames do not completely meet these requirements. If there are omissions or incorrect identification of elements, the effect is that the study population is less similar to the target population. If there is duplication, the duplicated elements have a higher probability of being selected, introducing a potential bias. An effort should be made to assess any potential sampling frame and to determine whether departures from the ideal are likely to introduce significant biases.

There are a number of approaches to randomization that can be used. Physical randomization involves the use of some physical random process to select from the sampling frame. Examples include rolling dice (particularly sets of decimal dice) or picking numbers on slips of paper from a bag. These methods are able to generate truly random numbers but can be very time consuming. They have the advantage, when done on-site, of clearly demonstrating to survey participants that the selection is random and that the inclusion or exclusion of individuals from the study is not happening for any intentional reason.

When a large sample is to be chosen, preprinted random number tables or computer-generated random numbers are usually more convenient. Random number tables are available in many statistical and epidemiological texts. EpiCalc 2000 (http://www.myatt.demon.co.uk/epicalc.htm) is freely available software that allows the simple generation of random numbers. (Strictly speaking, computers generate pseudorandom numbers, but the distinction is irrelevant for survey sampling purposes). If the sampling frame is available in the form of a computerized database, the Survey Toolbox software (http://www.ausvet.com.au/surveillance) contains a program to automatically select a sample from the sampling frame.

Selection from a sampling frame can be made with or without replacement. Sampling with replacement means that (conceptually) once an element has been chosen, it is then replaced in the population and has the chance of being chosen again. For large populations, there is little practical difference; however, as the population size decreases, it is important to know which approach is implemented. Sampling without replacement from small populations requires analysis using the hypergeometric distribution, whereas sampling with replacement uses the simpler binomial distribution.

Multistage sampling is an extension of simple random sampling. In multistage sampling, the population is divided into groups (e.g., cattle populations are naturally grouped into farms). The most common application of multistage sampling is two-stage sampling, although more stages can be used. In two-stage sampling, instead of constructing a sampling frame of all animals in the population, the first stage of sampling uses a sampling frame of all farms in the area. A random sample is chosen, and then sampling frames are constructed only for the selected farms. At the second stage, animals are chosen from these sampling frames. This system has the obvious advantage of removing the need for comprehensive sampling frames of large populations. It also reflects the clustered nature of the population. However, for a given sample size, estimates from two-stage sampling are less precise than those from simple random sampling.

One of the key limitations of simple random sampling (and, less so, two-stage sampling) is the requirement for a sampling frame. Random systematic sampling offers an approach to selecting an appropriate random sample in the absence of a sampling frame. This approach may be used if the population is able to be physically or notionally "lined up" in a sequence. The sample is selected by taking elements from that population at regular intervals. For example, a large flock of sheep may have no ear-tags or other individually identifying information. To generate a sampling frame, each sheep would first have to be identified. Instead, all sheep could be run through a race, and every tenth sheep (for example) could be selected for the sample. The sampling interval (in this example, 10) is calculated according to the following formula: $i = N/n$, where i is the sampling interval, N is the population size, and n is the desired sample size. The calculated interval is rounded down to an integer value.

Systematic sampling can be developed into random systematic sampling very simply. This involves random selection of the first animal by picking a random number between 1 and i, the sampling interval. After this first animal has been chosen at random, every i^{th} animal is selected for the rest of the sample. Random systematic sampling produces estimates that are essentially the same as simple random sampling, except in the unusual situation where the population being studied has cyclic variations that are synchronized with the sampling interval, in which case they may be biased.

Sampling Designs and Sample Size

Although sampling principles are essentially the same regardless of the objective of the survey or MOSS, the approach to calculating the sample size and methods of analysis differ depending on the objective. This section deals with sample size calculations for a number of common sampling designs for different survey types. The help menu for Win Episcope 2.0 (http://www.clive.ed.ac.uk/winepiscope) includes the relevant formulas.

Sample Size

Although different approaches are used to calculate sample size according to the survey objectives, the principles behind the calculation are the same in each case. A number of key pieces of information are required to calculate the sample size.

Maximum Tolerable Error of the Estimate
The maximum tolerable error of the estimate is how large an error we are willing to allow in our survey results; for example, ±5% (0.05). Other terms that are used for this measure include "bound on the error of estimation" or "error limits." For example, in a prevalence survey, we may feel that a result that is within ±10% of the true value is inadequate but that one that is within ±4% is adequate. Our desired maximum tolerable error for our survey estimate is, therefore, 4%.

Confidence
Confidence indicates the level of certainty that we have in our results and is, again, related to the confidence interval. By convention, a confidence level of 95% is used in most surveys, but other levels, for example, 90% or 99%, may also be used.

Power
Instead of simply estimating a quantity (such as an incidence or prevalence), some surveys or MOSS are designed to test hypotheses. Demonstrating freedom from disease is testing the hypothesis that disease prevalence is below some identified value. A prevalence survey may aim to determine whether prevalence has changed by more than a specified amount.

In these cases, the accuracy of a survey is measured in two ways: the power and the confidence. In hypothesis testing, a null hypothesis must first be established, usually meaning that there is no difference or no effect. In a comparison of two prevalence values, the null hypothesis would be that there is no real difference between the disease prevalence in the two populations. By convention, power is usually set to 80%, but this should be adjusted to take into account the consequences of failing to correctly identify a difference.

For hypothesis testing, software usually allows calculation of both a "one-tailed" and a "two-tailed" sample size. The choice of one-tail versus two-tail refers to the way in which the hypothesis is formulated. In a one-tailed test, we consider that a result in only one direction is of interest; for example, one value is less than another. A two-tailed test is used to determine whether one value is different to (either greater than or less than) another. Two-tailed sample sizes are larger than one-tailed sizes.

Variance
The variance measures the amount of variability in a characteristic in the population and has an important influence on sample size. This can be appreciated using an example: One study aims to find the mean weight of newborn piglets in a large pig herd. It is decided that a precision of ±200 g is acceptable. Almost all pigs born are within 200 g of the same weight, so no matter which piglets are selected, an estimate made on the basis of only a few is likely to be close to the true mean (and certainly within ±200 g). Therefore, only a very

small sample size is required, because the amount of variation in the population is small (relative to the desired precision).

Another study aims to find the mean weight of all pigs in the pig herd, and again uses a precision of ± 200 g. However, the weight of pigs varies from less than 1 kg up to hundreds of kilograms. There is a good chance that if only a few pigs were selected, the mean of their weights would not be very close to the overall herd mean. Instead, a very large number, perhaps almost all the pigs, would be required to estimate the mean weight and be within ± 200 g of the real value.

Understanding variance is one of the most challenging aspects to sample size calculations. In prevalence surveys, variance is related to the prevalence ($var = p\,(1 - p)$, where p is the prevalence). This means that to calculate the sample size required to estimate prevalence within a certain maximum tolerable error, an *a priori* estimate of prevalence is required. For proportions such as prevalence and cumulative incidence, the maximum variance occurs when $p = 0.5$, and hence, use of this value represents a worst-case scenario for sample size calculations. For two-stage sampling designs, the sample size calculations require input (prior estimates) about the variance between groups at each stage of sampling; for example, the amount of variation between herds and the amount of variation between animals within herds.

Population Size
The size of the population often has a small or negligible effect on sample size; variance is much more important. In most cases it can be ignored; however, sample sizes will decrease when the population size is small relative to the sample size. Increases in large population sizes (say from 10,000 to 100,000,000) generally have no effect on the sample size.

Test Accuracy
The accuracy of a test, measured by its sensitivity (probability that the result is positive given an animal is infected) and specificity (probability that the result is negative given an animal is noninfected), often has an influence on sample size calculations. When designing a study to detect disease or demonstrate freedom from disease, it is essential to take into account the effect of test accuracy.

For a sample size calculation to detect at least one truly positive animal in a herd, two values are necessary: desired confidence level (c) and the within-herd prevalence (p) of truly positive animals (Martin et al. 1992).

An approximation of the required sample size (n) $= \log(1 - c)/\log(1 - p)$. For example, assuming 95% confidence, the required sample size to detect a prevalence of 10% is 29 in an infinite population.

The formula above can be modified to include imperfect tests, in which case the new interpretation becomes the sample size needed to detect one test-positive animal at the specified level of confidence and disease prevalence.

The modified sample size is

$$n = \log(1 - c)/\{\log[Sp(1 - p) + (1 - Se)p]\},$$

where Se and Sp are sensitivity and specificity, respectively. Assume for the prior example that pathogen detection was by fecal culture, which has a sensitivity of 0.5 and specificity of 1. Substitution of these values yields a modified sample size of 58. This estimate could have been simply obtained by doubling the original sample size to adjust for the fact that only 50% of the diseased animals would be detected because of the tests lack of sensitivity. However, such simple adjustments can only easily be made when the test is perfectly specific. For tests that are imperfectly specific, the modified calculation must be used. For both formulas, it is possible to correct for finite population sizes, in which case the necessary sample size is smaller. Application of the finite population correction factor follows the same methods outlined for prevalence estimation as described in Chapter 5.

For prevalence surveys, however, while it is possible to incorporate test performance into sample size calculations, it is more usual to ignore the effect at the planning stage and to correct for imperfect test performance during data analysis. However, the choice not to consider the uncertainty in test accuracy in the planning phase often results in less precise prevalence estimates than expected.

Prevalence and Incidence

The commonly used (approximate) formula for calculating sample size for a prevalence survey is based on the normal approximation to the binomial distribution, and it has as inputs maximum tolerable error (L), confidence level ($1 - \alpha$), estimated prevalence (p), and population size (N).

The approximate formula for the sample size (n) is

$$n = \left(\frac{Z_\alpha}{L}\right)^2 p(1 - p),$$

where Z_α is the tabulated Z value for the desired level of confidence (ie, 1.96 when $\alpha = 0.05$). To calculate the adjusted sample size (n_c) for finite population sizes, the following formula may be used.

$$n_c = \frac{n}{1 + \frac{n}{N}}.$$

For an estimated $p = 0.5$ with a maximum error of ± 0.1 and 95% confidence, the calculated value of n is 96 in an infinite population. Assuming that the total population size was 200, the adjusted sample size (n_c)$= 96/(1 + 96/200) \approx 65$.

These calculations are implemented in a number of free software packages, including Win Episcope 2.0 and EpiCalc 2000.

Calculation of sample sizes for comparing two prevalences (e.g., when running a MOSS that aims to detect changes in prevalence over time) requires a slightly different approach. This is because of the difference between estimating a single value (prevalence in a study population) and testing a hypothesis (that two prevalence estimates are different). The sample size calculation can be done in the same programs. The inputs required are estimated prevalence in the first population (p_1), estimated prevalence in the second population (p_2), confidence level$(1 - \alpha)$, and power $(1 - \beta)$.

The required sample size is

$$ n = \left(\frac{Z_\alpha + Z_\beta}{p_1 - p_2} \right) [p_1(1 - p_1) + p_2(1 - p_2)], $$

where Z_α is tabulated Z value for the desired level of confidence $(1 - \alpha)$ and Z_β is the Z value for the desired power $(1 - \beta)$.

The same formulas can be used for sample size calculations for incidence studies in which cumulative incidence is the risk measure of interest.

Mean

In a MOSS, sometimes the key outcome of interest is the mean value of a characteristic that is measured on a continuous scale and either change in population means over time or differences of means between populations are assessed. For example, monitoring the effect of a selenium supplementation program may be achieved by assessing mean selenium concentrations in blood at regular intervals. The approach to calculating sample size for such a study is very similar to that used for prevalence. In fact, prevalence can be thought of as exactly the same as the mean, where positive animals have a value of 1 and negative animals have a value of 0. The inputs for the calculation are desired error limit (d), confidence level $(1 - \alpha)$, population size (N), and variation of the outcome of interest in the population, which is usually expressed in terms of the standard deviation (SD). This must be estimated based on previous studies or a pilot study.

$$ n = \left(\frac{SD(Z_\alpha)}{d} \right)^2. $$

The finite population correction shown above for prevalence estimation can be applied to the result.

For hypothesis testing (determining whether two means are statistically different), the inputs are again similar to those used for prevalence surveys: estimated mean in the first population, x_1; estimated mean in the second population (indicating the magnitude of change that is to be detected), x_2; SD (in simple formulas, assumed to be constant between the two samples); confidence level $(1 - \alpha)$; and power $(1 - \beta)$.

The required sample size is:

$$n = \left(\frac{SD(Z_\alpha + Z_\beta)}{\bar{x}_1 - \bar{x}_2} \right)^2.$$

Freedom from Disease or Detection of Disease

Surveys to demonstrate freedom from disease (or in the case of an infectious agent, freedom from the specific pathogen) are examples of hypothesis testing studies. The factors that need to be considered when calculating sample size are confidence level $(1 - \alpha)$, power $(1 - \beta)$, test performance (sensitivity and specificity), population size, and minimum detectable prevalence.

No survey is able to guarantee that a population is free from disease. If a sample is used, it is always possible that a very small number of (or even a single) diseased animals exists in the population and was not selected in the sample. Even if the entire population were tested, imperfect sensitivity means that any positive animal may have given a negative test result. This survey approach therefore does not attempt to prove absolute freedom. Instead, the survey determines the probability of observing a given number of reactors (test-positive animals), based on random sampling, from sample of size n from a population that is diseased at a specified prevalence. If the probability is small, we can be confident that the disease, if present in the study population, has a prevalence less than that specified to calculate the sample size. Depending on the nature of the disease and the selected threshold prevalence, this may be widely accepted as proof of freedom. For instance, it is extremely unlikely that a highly contagious or fatal disease would have a very low prevalence in a naïve population. In other cases, disease may be present at low prevalence, but it is either impractical to detect it or so economically or biologically unimportant at those levels as to not warrant the effort to determine its "true" prevalence.

The FreeCalc program in Survey Toolbox can perform the calculation of sample size, and the formula used is described in Cameron and Baldock (1998a) and shown subsequently in "Sample Size."

SPECIAL SAMPLING SITUATIONS

Pooled Samples

Pooling of samples involves combining a number of specimens and testing them together. Examples include pooled fecal culture, in which a number of fecal samples from different animals is mixed and cultured, and bulk milk testing, in which a sample of bulk milk is tested rather than samples from individual cows. The theory behind using pooled samples is that if one or more animals in the pool are positive, the pool will be positive. If all are negative, then the pool will be negative. The advantage of using pooled samples is that specimens from many animals can be screened using a single test, thereby saving time and money, especially if the pooling procedure is not labor intensive and prevalence is low. There are, however, a number of considerations that must be taken into account. The most obvious disadvantage is that the results of the test can no longer be directly related to individual specimens. If a pool reacts positively, it means that at least one of the component specimens is positive. To determine which individuals are positive, the individual specimens that went into the positive pool must be separately tested. If multiple pools are tested from a population, it also is possible to estimate individual animal prevalence from the pooled test results. The approach of testing pools and then retesting individual specimens in positive pools can save a considerable amount of testing, but this depends on the balance between pool size (number of specimens per pool) and prevalence. It is most efficient with low-prevalence diseases, with which only a small number of pools needs to be retested. With larger pools, the more likely it is that a pool will need to be retested, but the lower the initial costs. Small pools have higher initial testing costs, but a lower chance of requiring retesting.

The relationship between pool size (x) and prevalence (p) below which pooled testing is cost effective is given by the equation

$$p < 1 - x\sqrt{\tfrac{1}{x}}.$$

The maximum prevalence below which a pool of known size is cost effective is shown in Table 4.1.

Pooled samples may also be used to determine the status of a group of animals instead of individual animals as in the example above (i.e., as a herd test). In this case, it is not necessary to retest individual specimens if a pool is positive.

In both situations, there is a practical limitation to the maximum size of the pool, which is related to the ability of the test to detect positive specimens when diluted by a number of negative specimens. The sensitivity of the pooled test of fixed size should be comparable to the sensitivity of the test on an individual sample if one wants to estimate individual prevalence. Before use in a MOSS, the pooled test should be evaluated to determine its ability to identify single positive samples in pools of differing sizes and to determine its sensitivity and specificity under these conditions.

Continuous Populations

Not all populations can be described as a collection of discrete elements, such as farms or animals. Instead, they are made up of a continuous substance. Examples include sampling air or water for environmental contaminants or sampling feed for pathogens and toxins. Despite these differences, the same types

TABLE 4.1   Maximum Prevalence Below Which a Pool of Known Size Is Cost Effective

Pool size	Maximum prevalence	Pool size	Maximum prevalence	Pool size	Maximum prevalence
3	0.307	24	0.124	45	0.081
4	0.293	25	0.121	46	0.080
5	0.275	26	0.118	47	0.079
6	0.258	27	0.115	48	0.077
7	0.243	28	0.112	49	0.076
8	0.229	29	0.110	50	0.075
9	0.217	30	0.107	51	0.074
10	0.206	31	0.105	52	0.073
11	0.196	32	0.103	53	0.072
12	0.187	33	0.101	54	0.071
13	0.179	34	0.099	55	0.070
14	0.172	35	0.097	56	0.069
15	0.165	36	0.095	57	0.068
16	0.159	37	0.093	58	0.068
17	0.154	38	0.091	59	0.067
18	0.148	39	0.090	60	0.066
19	0.144	40	0.088	61	0.065
20	0.139	41	0.087	62	0.064
21	0.132	42	0.085	63	0.064
22	0.131	43	0.084	64	0.063
23	0.127	44	0.082		

of sampling strategies can be applied by artificially dividing the substance to be sampled into discrete units. This can be illustrated by a few examples: A study aims to examine a prepared pelleted feed for the presence of a bacterial contaminant. Samples are to be collected at the factory. The target population may be the feed produced by the factory, but the study must be limited to feed produced during a certain period of time. In the factory, feed is transported via an auger for bagging, and specimens are collected for examination as the feed enters the bags. This situation is ideal for systematic random sampling, as the whole population is lined up and can be sampled at regular intervals. The interval can be measured in terms of bags (e.g., a sample is taken from every tenth bag being filled) or, if the flow of feed during production is constant, it can be measured in terms of time (a sample is taken every 10 minutes). Random systematic sampling can be achieved by randomly selecting the bag or time of the first sample.

A study is conducted to assess air quality in large ships used to transport cattle. The objective is to assess the mean value of a number of indicators, including temperature, humidity, dust, and ammonia, and their maximum and variability. The population needs to be defined in a number of dimensions: It consists of all the air in the cattle-carrying compartments of the ship during the period of the voyage. Previous studies have used data-logging equipment, located at a number of fixed points distributed throughout the ship, to sample the air several times a day (e.g., at 9:00 AM and 6:00 PM). This approach may produce biased results, as the locations selected may not be truly representative and the sampling times are synchronized with diurnal variations. An improved approach would be to select a random sample, in both time and space. To select a random sample in time, the total period of the voyage is estimated in minutes, and this is used as the "temporal population," from which n random times are chosen. Second, the dimensions of the ship are measured, and sets of three random numbers are generated, describing the spatial x, y, and z coordinates of each sampling location. These are matched with the random times (in the same order as they were selected) to create a truly random sample of the air during the voyage.

This type of approach may be adapted to a wide range of situations and dimensions. A single dimension may be used to sample along a line (e.g., a stock transport route). Two dimensions may be used for an area (soil samples on a farm), three for a volume (water in a tank), or four if time is also included.

Sampling Without a Sampling Frame—Proxy Sampling

Simple random sampling and the probability sampling schemes that are derived from it require a sampling frame. Random systematic sampling removes this need but can only be used when the population can be lined up in some fashion. There are many situations in which no reliable sampling frame is available and the population cannot be lined up. One example is the problem of sampling wildlife. One approach that may be used in these situations is proxy sampling. In proxy sampling, instead of selecting the sampling elements themselves (e.g., animals), something else is selected as a proxy for the elements (e.g., spatial locations). The randomly selected proxies are then associated with the elements (e.g., by identifying the animal nearest the random location).

Proxy sampling works most effectively when there is a reliable one-to-one relationship between the element and the proxy. When this is not the case (e.g., many spatial locations without nearby animals and some locations with a number of animals nearby), special care needs to be taken to avoid introducing biases into the sample.

CONCLUSION

The design of an effective survey or MOSS is dependent on a number of considerations that have been described in Chapter 1 and 2. From a statistical viewpoint, a key issue is the selection of an appropriate sampling technique and sample size to meet the specified objectives. Analysis methods and inference follow logically from the chosen design. In this chapter, we described sampling methods and sample size calculations.

BIBLIOGRAPHY

Cameron A.R., and Baldock F.C. 1998a. A new probability formula for surveys to substantiate freedom from disease. Prev Vet Med 34:1–17.

Christensen J., Gardner I.A. 2000. Herd-level interpretation of diagnostic tests. Prev Vet Med 45:83–106.

Martin S.W., Shoukri M., Thorburn M.A. 1992. Evaluating the health status of herds based on tests applied to individuals. Prev Vet Med 75:596–600.

Chapter 5

Statistical Analysis of Data from Surveys, Monitoring, and Surveillance Systems

B. Wagner,[1] I. Gardner,[2] A. Cameron,[3] and M.G. Doherr[4]

SINGLE SURVEY APPROACHES

Surveys intended to evaluate disease prevalence (p) over a wide geographic region or an entire country require a practical sampling approach that accounts for the occurrence of animals in groups or clusters such as herds or flocks. Cluster or two-stage sampling can be used as a strategy to investigate disease prevalence among groups of animals. The primary sampling unit in these types of sampling is the cluster; for example, a herd. In cluster sampling, all the units within a cluster are sampled, whereas with two-stage sampling, only a selected subset of the units in a cluster is sampled. Clusters can be selected by simple

[1]USDA:APHIS:VS:CEAH, Mail Stop #2E7, 2150 Centre Avenue, Building B, Fort Collins, CO 80526–8117

[2]Department of Medicine and Epidemiology, School of Veterinary Medicine, University of California, Davis, CA 95616

[3]Ausvet Animal Health Services, Wentworth Falls, New South Wales 2782, Australia

[4]Department of Veterinary Clinical Medicine, University of Bern, Bern, Switzerland CH-3001

random sampling or be subject to a more complex design such as a stratified random sample.

In the context of a monitoring and surveillance system (MOSS), sampling of clusters has some inherent advantages over other sampling designs. First, random sampling of clusters requires only a list of herds or flocks rather than a list of individual animal elements. A list frame of operations (e.g., farms) for a large geographic area can be built and maintained, but it would be very difficult and expensive to construct a list of individual elements (animals). Second, one of the objectives of MOSS activities might be to estimate both cluster- and animal-level prevalence. Sampling clusters allows for estimation at both levels and for consideration of both herd- and animal-level factors that may influence health and production (McDermott and Schukken 1994). Finally, cluster (or two-stage) sampling allows for adjusting the sampling protocol according to the degree of similarity of the individuals within a cluster. The similarity among individuals in a cluster may arise from factors such as the influence of common management practices or from exposure and transmission of infectious agents.

INTRACLUSTER CORRELATION COEFFICIENT

The measure of the congregation of diseased (or healthy) animals within a cluster is referred to as the intracluster correlation coefficient (ICC; Donald 1993; McDermott and Schukken 1994). The ICC, ρ, has a value between 0 and 1. If $\rho = 0$, then the disease is randomly distributed within a population and animals from within a herd are no more likely to be diseased than any animal selected from the entire population. When $\rho = 1$, then all animals within a herd have the same status. Thus, when using cluster sampling, as ρ approaches 1, the herd is behaving more like an individual, and fewer animals within a herd would need to be evaluated to determine herd status. Under this scenario, more herds and fewer animals per herd would be an appropriate sampling strategy. When ρ is close to 0, then animals are behaving as if they were randomly distributed throughout the population, and it may be more appropriate to sample more animals per herd and fewer herds to optimize the design. McDermott and Schukken (1994) reviewed a number of papers from the veterinary epidemiology literature and found that, where estimable, ρ varied between 0.0017 and 0.46.

When only two sampling levels are being examined (e.g., a herd and animals within a herd), one approach to calculation of the ICC is to use the analysis of variance (ANOVA) estimator (Donner and Donald 1987). The value is estimated by

$$\rho = \frac{(MSB - MSW)}{(MSB + n - 1) \times MSW}$$

where MSB is the between cluster mean square, MSW is the within cluster mean square, and n is the mean cluster size. Ridout et al. (1999) provide a detailed review of methods for estimating ρ. In situations in which the cluster size (n) is highly variable, the ANOVA estimator for the ICC may not always perform adequately.

ANIMAL- AND HERD-LEVEL PREVALENCE ESTIMATION

Estimation Based on the Assumption of Perfect Diagnostic Testing

Estimation of prevalence and associated variances can be very complex in large-scale veterinary epidemiologic studies. The clustering of animals within herds may affect the variance estimate for the animal-level analysis. Sensitivity and specificity of the test being used to evaluate animals can have a profound effect on the animal- and herd-level estimates. We have chosen the example of Johne's disease to demonstrate the methods and the effect of design and test characteristics on the estimation process.

In 1996, the National Animal Health Monitoring System conducted a study of the U.S. dairy industry and focused a portion of the study on Johne's disease (Wells and Wagner 2000). Johne's disease is a chronic disease of ruminants caused by the slow-growing bacterium *Mycobacterium avian paratuberculosis* (*M. paratuberculosis*). A stratified random sample of dairy herds with at least 30 milking cows was selected from 20 states of the United States. The within-herd sampling protocol was designed to detect at least 1 seropositive cow with 90% confidence assuming a prevalence of at least 5% in herds and a test sensitivity and specificity of 45% and 99%, respectively. The protocol specified collecting sera from 25 cows from herds with 30 to 49 cows, 30 cows from herds with 50 to 99 cows, 35 cows from herds with 100 to 299 cows, and 40 cows from herds with 300 or more cows. The sample included 31,745 cows from 977 herds that were tested for antibodies to *M. paratuberculosis*. Herds that had vaccinated for *M. paratuberculosis* were excluded from the analysis.

A total of 789 of the 31,745 cows were test positive ($\hat{p} = 0.025$ or 2.5%). Assuming a perfect diagnostic test and an independent random sample, even though the design was two-stage within a stratified random sample, the appropriate variance is

$$V_p = \frac{\hat{p}(1 - \hat{p})}{n},$$

where $\hat{p}$ is the estimated proportion. The estimated variance is 0.000001 (standard error = 0.0009). Although $\hat{p}$ is an unbiased estimate, the variance is likely biased downward because the independence assumption is violated. Using a normal approximation, the 95% confidence interval is 0.025 ± 1.96 × 0.0009 (95% confidence interval = 0.023 to 0.027). Exact binomial confidence intervals can be used as an alternative to the normal approximation to the binomial distribution and are preferred when the normal approximation is inappropriate (Blyth 1986).

In the situation where disease prevalence is rare (<10%) and the objective is to estimate animal-level prevalence, pooling of samples offers an economic alternative method of testing. Cowling et al. (1999) described three methods for estimating prevalence and associated variance under the assumption of a perfect diagnostic test. They also provided two methods, a continuity-correction and an exact method, for determining confidence intervals.

The ICC can be used to adjust the variance for the lack of independence within clusters (Donald and Donner 1987). The variance correction factor,

$$C = 1 + (n - 1) \times \hat{\rho},$$

incorporates the ICC to inflate the variance. Using the ANOVA method, the intracluster correlation coefficient for these data was 0.04, which indicated minimal clustering of disease. This result is reflected in the distribution of positive test results. In 91.6% of the herds tested, there were either one or zero positive test results. Only 3% of the herds had four or more positive test results. The adjusted variance is 0.000002 (standard error = 0.0013). The 95% confidence interval with the adjusted variance is 0.022 to 0.028.

The National Animal Health Monitoring System uses SUDAAN software (version 8.0; Research Triangle Institute, Research Triangle Park, NC) to estimate variance. SUDAAN has implemented a Taylor series expansion estimate of variance, which accounts for the clustering and the stratified random design. The variance estimate from SUDAAN for the Johne's data was 0.000003 (standard error = 0.0017). The 95% confidence interval (0.022 to 0.028) is similar to the interval obtained with the variance inflation correction.

Estimation of herd-level prevalence, under the assumption of perfect testing, is straightforward. Herd status can be defined as positive if a single positive individual test or a positive pooled test occurs in the herd. The herd-level prevalence and standard error could then be computed based on the design (simple random sample or stratified random sample). However, the sampling design for the Johne's study was based on detecting, with a specified probability, a positive herd if the prevalence was greater than 5% given imperfect test sensitivity and specificity. The sampling strategy likely will result in herd misclassification based on both the sampling intensity and the test accuracy. Even if the issue of imperfect test performance is ignored, herd prevalence can be calculated, but the inference should reflect the sampling intensity.

A total of 413 herds ($p = 0.423$ or 42.3%) had at least one positive test. Assuming a simple random sample, the resulting 95% confidence interval based on a normal approximation to the binomial is 0.39 to 0.45. The inference should reflect that (again assuming a perfect test) the prevalence is for herds with 5% prevalence or higher. If the inference is assumed to be for all positive herds, then the estimate is likely downwardly biased. The bias is introduced because diseased herds may not be detected when the sample selected for testing does not include diseased animals. Given the within-herd sampling protocol, herds with 5% prevalence can be misclassified (5% of the time because of the stated confidence), but the misclassification rate will likely be even higher with herds that have prevalence lower than 5%. The bias is again introduced because there is a probability that the reduced number of positive animals in the herd will not be included in the tested sample. If the sample size comprises more than 5% of population size, the sensitivity of the sampling strategy can be explored using the hypergeometric distribution. If the sample size is less than 5% of the population size, then the binomial distribution will give a reasonable approximation of the hypergeometric distribution.

Estimation Based on Imperfect Diagnostic Testing

Both animal- and herd-level apparent prevalences will be biased estimates of the true prevalence if an imperfect diagnostic test is used. If sensitivity (Se) and specificity (Sp) are known, then estimates of apparent prevalence can be adjusted. If Se and Sp are unknown, then distributional attributes may be derived but either Bayesian or simulation models will be necessary to account for this uncertainty.

Rogan and Gladen (1978) presented an estimator of true prevalence if Se and Sp are known and fixed:

$$p_{rg} = \frac{\hat{p} + Sp - 1}{Se + Sp - 1}.$$

The procedure for adjusting the prevalence will affect the variance. Greiner and Gardner (2000) showed that variation is essentially $1/J^2$ times the variance of the original variance, where $J = Se + Sp - 1$. If we assume a 45% Se and a 99% Sp for the enzyme-linked immunosorbent assay (ELISA) used in the Johne's study, then we can adjust the animal-level prevalence and its associated variance. The true prevalence estimate for the Johne's study is 3.4%. The variance increased fivefold to 0.000005, which substantially increases the 95% confidence interval (0.030 to 0.038). If Se and Sp are assumed to be constants, then the same adjustment could be made to the variance estimates obtained using either the variance inflation factor or the Taylor's series expansion. If Se and Sp are unknown, the uncertainty can be accounted for by using a Taylor's series expansion that has been developed for use when the observations can be considered to be independent (Greiner and Gardner 2000).

Pooled sampling approaches can also be considered even when the diagnostic tests are imperfect and when the disease being estimated is rare. The precision of estimates can be comparable to those of individual sample testing if the sensitivity of pooled testing is equivalent to that of the individual test (Cowling et al. 1999). Cowling et al. (1999) described methods for estimating animal-level prevalence and associated confidence intervals using pools when the sensitivity and specificity are known and have fixed values. In veterinary medicine applications, the diagnostic test characteristics are often unknown and typically are considered fixed values to apply to all populations. Cowling et al. (1999) presented an example of eggs contaminated with *Salmonella enteritidis* to demonstrate frequentist and Bayesian approaches to estimating individual-level prevalence from pooled samples when sensitivity and specificity are unknown.

Herd-level prevalence estimation must account for potential misclassification attributable to sampling error and imperfect diagnostic tests (individual or pooled). Cameron and Baldock (1998a) presented the idea that a screening test applied to animals within a cluster with the purpose of classifying the cluster as diseased or nondiseased is essentially a herd-level test with its own S_e and S_p. The herd-level S_e and S_p are determined largely by the number of test-positive animals that are needed to classify the cluster as positive. As the number of test-positive animals increases, the S_e decreases and the S_p increases. They presented a modification of the hypergeometric formula to calculate the exact probability of observing a specific number of test positives given the cluster size, sample size, and known S_e and S_p.

$$P(T^+ = x) = \sum_{y=0}^{d} \frac{\binom{d}{y}\binom{N-d}{n-y}}{\binom{N}{n}} \sum_{j=0}^{min(x,y)} \binom{y}{j} Se^j (1 - Se)^{y-j}$$

$$\times \binom{n-y}{x-j}(1 - Sp)^{x-j} Sp^{n-x-y+j},$$

where T^+ is the number of test positives, d is the number of diseased animals, N is the population size, and n is the sample size. The hypergeometric distribution accounts for the probability of selecting a diseased animal in a sample from a finite population. A computer implementation of the formula is available in the Freecalc software developed by Cameron (http://epiweb.massey .ac.nz/ or (http://www.ausvet.com.au/surveillance).

The Johne's disease study exemplifies some of the complexities involved with using this approach to determine herd-level test characteristics. Herd and sample sizes varied, necessitating a computation of herd-level sensitivity (HSE) and specificity (HSP) for each combination. For example, when 30 samples are taken from a herd of 50 animals (S_e = 45% and S_p = 99%), a minimum expected prevalence of 5% and a cut point of one positive to declare the herd positive results in a HSE of 60% and a HSP of 74%. If the herd size is 200 and a sample of 35 animals is taken, the HSE is 69% and the HSP is 70%. We are unaware of a nonmodeling approach that would allow for combination of these variable HSE and HSP values. We emphasize that these calculations of HSE and HSP assume that estimates of individual-level test sensitivity and specificity are unbiased. If individual estimates are biased, the bias in HSE and HSP will be much greater than at the individual level (Christensen and Gardner 2000).

A different approach was taken to calculate herd-level prevalence in the Johne's study. A cut-off point of two positives was required to define a herd as positive (U.S. Department of Agriculture [USDA] 1997). This alone would increase the HSP to 95% but decrease the HSE to 31% (N = 200, n = 35). The HSE was increased by allowing inclusion of herds with a single test-positive animal and a questionnaire response that indicated clinical signs of Johne's disease in at least 5% of cull cows. Although this approach allowed for estimation of herd-level prevalence (21.6%), it was not possible to estimate the final HSE and HSP. The variance was computed assuming that the true herd status had been assessed with the testing protocol using the normal approximation to the binomial distribution.

BAYESIAN ANALYSIS

Bayesian methods are currently being evaluated as an alternative approach to traditional statistical methods (Cameron and Baldock 1998b; Martin et al. 1992) and simulation modeling (Audigé and Beckett 1999) for the analysis of herd-level test results and population surveys (Audigé et al. 2001).

The Bayesian approach allows the analyst to combine prior data or expert opinion about prevalence and test accuracy with current herd-level test results (usually termed the likelihood) to produce updated posterior inferences about within-herd prevalence and the proportion of infected herds. For complicated analyses, Gibbs sampling (an iterative Markov-chain Monte-Carlo simulation method; Casella and George 1992; Robert and Casella 1999) is needed to obtain these outputs.

The primary advantage of Bayesian methods over traditional statistical methods is that uncertainty in each parameter is modeled as a probability distribution and, thus, the posterior distributions that are obtained in the analysis can be used to calculate 95% credible intervals for within-herd prevalence and the proportion of infected herds. In contrast to confidence intervals, credible intervals have a direct probabilistic interpretation. Bayesian approaches also do not result in negative prevalence estimates, as can sometimes occur with traditional adjustment methods (Rogan and Gladen 1978). The major criticism of Bayesian methods is that the prior may have a strong effect on the posterior distribution as the posterior is essentially a weighted average of the prior and the data. Solutions to this problem are to use uniform or noninformative priors as input or for the investigator to do a sensitivity analysis using different priors to evaluate the effects on model outputs.

Prior Distributions

For prevalence surveys, most of the inputs are binomial event probabilities (e.g., test sensitivity and specificity and the proportion of infected herds). Beta distributions are a suitable choice to model such probabilities because beta distribution is the most appropriate distribution for binomial data, and the distribution is restricted to values between 0 and 1 (Vose 1996). One method of constructing a beta distribution is to use data from previous studies. For example, if a previous test-evaluation study involved the testing of 14 infected animals and 7 animals tested positive and 7 animals tested negative, then a beta (8, 8) distribution as shown in Figure 5.1 would be appropriate for modeling sensitivity estimate of 50%.

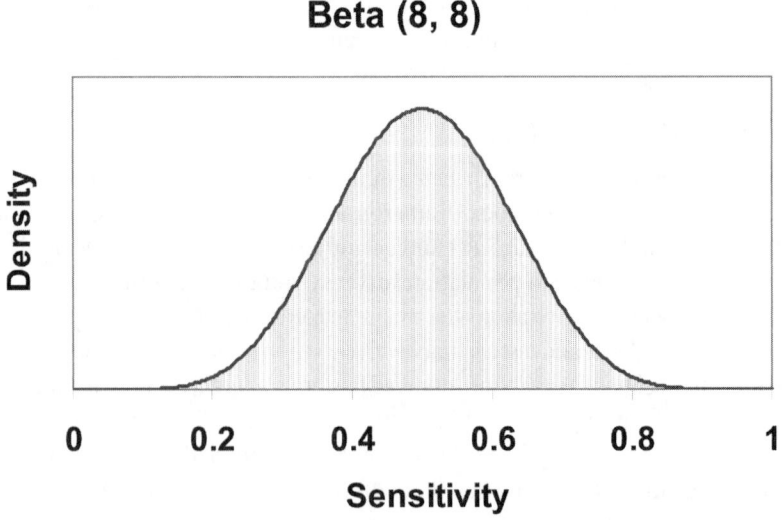

FIGURE 5.1   A beta (8,8) probability distribution can be used to model a sensitivity estimate of 50% that is based on test results of 14 infected animals.

In general, if an experiment resulted in s successes (e.g., number of test-positive animals) recorded in n trials (e.g., number of truly infected animals), use of a beta (a, b) distribution with $a = s + 1$ and $b = n - s + 1$ is an appropriate choice to model the uncertainty in that parameter. Alternatively, one can elicit expert opinion about a binomial parameter by asking for the best currently available estimate (which is equated to the mode of the beta $[a, b]$ distribution) and also asking for an interval in which the expert strongly believes the true value to lie. If the upper and lower end points of the interval are taken to be the 5th and 95th percentage points of a corresponding beta distribution, it is straightforward to find appropriate values for a and b (see Suess et al. 2002 for details). The corresponding beta density is drawn and verified by the expert. In the absence of such prior data, or to ascertain the effect of the selected prior distribution on the posterior distribution, noninformative priors (e.g., beta [1, 1] distributions) are used.

Two-stage Cluster Surveys

A hierarchical model that analyzes herd-level test results has been developed and is currently being assessed for disease freedom certification and for analysis of survey data for endemic diseases from multiple herds. In the model, three levels of inference are possible: country, herd, and animal. The model has been validated with simulated data and has been used to assess freedom from Newcastle disease (ND) virus in Swiss laying hens and freedom from porcine reproductive and respiratory syndrome virus in Swiss pigs (Suess et al. 2002). Because of the complexity of the analysis, Gibbs sampling is needed to obtain a solution. Details of these analyses are given in the following sections.

Newcastle Disease

In 1996, blood samples were collected at a central poultry slaughterhouse from 30 birds in 260 Swiss egg-laying flocks (Gohm et al. 1999). Sera were tested for antibodies to ND by ELISA. Most flocks were negative ($n = 194$) or had a low number of test-positive birds ($n = 62$), but four flocks had many reactors (10, 10, 14, and 22, repsectively). Prior estimates (most likely values and ranges) were elicited from an expert for test accuracy, the proportion of infected flocks, and within-flock prevalence before doing the survey, as described in the previous section. Updated posterior distributions of within-flock prevalence and the proportion of infected flocks were obtained as outputs from the analysis. At each iteration of the model, a latent variable ($Z = 0$ or 1) was generated that indicated whether Switzerland had ND (1) or was free of ND (0). In the analysis, all $Z = 1$, which indicated that Swiss poultry had ND at the time of the survey. In Table 5.1, prior and posterior probabilities (modes and 95% intervals) are shown.

Although usually not of primary interest, updated estimates of sensitivity and specificity were obtained as additional model outputs. The estimate of the

TABLE 5.1   Bayesian Analysis of Newcastle Disease in 260 Swiss laying flocks

Parameter	Prior mode	Prior 95% interval	Posterior mode	Posterior 95% interval
Within-flock prevalence	0.3	0.16 to 0.50	0.39	0.27 to 0.51
Proportion of infected flocks	0.01	0.002 to 0.059	0.018	0.007 to 0.035
ELISA sensitivity	0.995	0.965 to 0.999	0.995	0.967 to 0.999
ELISA specificity	0.995	0.977 to 0.999	0.990	0.988 to 0.992

Note. Based on Gohm et al. 1999.

Abbreviation: ELISA, enzyme-linked immunosorbent assay.

proportion of infected flocks increased from a prior estimate of 0.01 to 0.018, reflecting the finding that four (1.5%) of 260 flocks had a substantial number of reactors. The posterior distribution of the proportion of infected flocks was narrower than the prior distribution because of the large number of flocks that had negative test results.

Porcine Reproductive and Respiratory Syndrome Virus
A serologic survey for PRRS was done in 1996 to verify that Swiss pigs were free of the virus (Canon et al. 1998). Five pigs in each of 108 herds were sampled, and all 540 samples were negative on the PRRS ELISA. Prior distributions were elicited from an expert for test accuracy, the proportion of infected herds, and within-herd prevalence, as previously described. The posterior analysis indicated that the country was not infected and that the mode for the proportion of infected herds was 0.017 compared with the prior mode of 0.05. Posterior inferences were not possible about within-herd prevalence because all the test results were negative.

Findings from both analyses were similar to those obtained by simulation modeling. The major advantage of the Bayesian method over simulation modeling for these data was that it yielded updated distributions for the proportion of infected herds (both diseases) and within-herd prevalence (ND only). Distributions of the proportion of infected flocks and within-flock prevalence are useful for risk analysts involved in trade decisions.

SIMULATION MODELING

Simulation models provide an alternative approach to estimation of herd- and animal-level prevalence. Uncertainty in underlying parameters such as the intracluster correlation for variation in prevalence among herd, sensitivity, and specificity can be incorporated into the model, and software to implement these modifications has been written (Jordan and McEwen 1998). A more detailed discussion of simulation modeling is included in Chapter 11.

REPEATED SURVEY APPROACHES

In this section, we consider analysis of repeated surveys, which are done as part of national surveys to document disease freedom and also as part of a MOSS to monitor success of disease eradication programs. In addition, repeated herd testing is done during surveillance of specific-pathogen-free (SPF) swine herds for important respiratory pathogens (Sørensen et al. 1992) or sentinel cattle herds for vector-borne diseases such as bluetongue (Ward et al. 1995).

At a national level, different herds almost always are involved in the testing, but on a smaller scale (e.g., SPF programs and sentinel herds); the same herds (but sometimes different animals within those herds) are retested. As for single surveys, a critical issue is the choice of an appropriate threshold (number of test-positive results) to designate the herd a positive (Martin et al. 1992).

Methods of analysis and confidence interval calculation follow those for single surveys. In addition to true and apparent herd prevalence, it might be possible to calculate true and apparent herd-level cumulative incidence providing that the same herds are tested in the two surveys. Similarly, at an individual animal level, cumulative incidence or incidence density rates and 95% confidence intervals can be calculated if the same individual animals are retested in herds. On the basis of a review of the published veterinary literature, we were unable to find incidence estimates corrected for intracluster correlation when two-stage sampling designs were used.

Specific-pathogen-free Swine Herds

The SPF program for Danish pig herds was established in 1968 to minimize the risk of dissemination of important pathogens including *Mycoplasma hyopneumoniae* and *Actinobacillus pleuropneumoniae*, which are commonly associated with conventional pig herds. Approximately 3,500 herds are involved in the program including about 120 breeding and multiplying herds (Sørensen et al. 1992, 1993). These latter herds are monitored by monthly clinical inspections. In addition, 20 blood samples are taken and analyzed for antibodies to *M. hyopneumoniae* and *A. pleuropneumoniae* by ELISA. Necropsies and occasional slaughterhouse checks are done to complement clinical and serologic monitoring for pathogens. SPF programs in pig herds in other countries use similar procedures.

The risk of reintroduction of *M. hyopneumoniae* into 124 SPF breeding and multiplying herds during 1990 was studied by Sørensen et al. (1992). Eighteen (14.5%) of 124 herds became reinfected over a 6-month period based on culture and identification of the organism. Using two serologic tests, an indirect hemagglutination test and a competitive ELISA, estimates of apparent herd incidence rates were 20 (16.1%) of 124 and 18 (14.9%) of 121, respectively. The criterion for designating the herd as positive was at least one positive serum sample out of 20 on either IHA or ELISA. Although not reported in the paper, 95% confidence intervals for these proportions can be calculated by exact binomial methods or approximate methods. Exact 95% confidence intervals for true and apparent herd incidence were 8.8% to 22.0% (true), 10.1% to 23.8% (IHA), and 9.1% to 22.5% (ELISA).

During 1991, a follow-up study of 134 SPF breeding and multiplying herds was done (Sørensen et al. 1993). The annual herd-level incidence of *M. hyopneumoniae* was 9.7% (95% confidence interval = 5.2% to 16.0%) based on confirmation by culturing and identification of the agent. Apparent herd-level incidence of *M. hyopneumoniae* was based on ELISA results. Two criteria were used for classification of the herds on the basis of ELISA results: at least one positive or at least two positive versus zero or one positive. On the basis of these criteria, 31 (23.1%: 95% confidence interval = 16.3 to 31.2%) and 13 (9.7%; 95% confidence interval = 5.2 to 16.0%) herds, respectively, were considered positive.

Sentinel Cattle Herds for Arboviral Infections

In Australia, a sentinel herd scheme was developed during the 1970s with the primary purpose of enabling the isolation and identification of arboviruses, especially bluetongue viruses that had not been previously found in northern regions of Australia (Gard et al. 1988). Serologic testing of sentinel cattle was done with the agar-gel immunodiffusion (AGID) test for group-specific bluetongue antibodies, and positive AGID samples were followed with serotype-specific serum neutralization (SN) tests. Between 10 and 20 cattle negative to the AGID test and aged about 6 to 9 months were randomly selected in each sentinel herd for follow-up testing. Cattle usually were sampled monthly during the follow-up period.

Between 1990 and 1992, Ward et al. (1995) evaluated seroconversion to bluetongue virus (defined as an SN titer of ≥1:20 in an animal that was previously negative) in 498 cattle in 47 herds monitored in Queensland, Australia. Of 498 cattle, 78 (15.7%) seroconverted to serotype 1 or serotype 21. These seroconversions occurred in 16 (34.0%) of 47 herds.

Because follow-up periods were not identical for all herds and some animals were lost to follow-up, incidence density rates (IDRs) were calculated as the preferred method of comparing among-herd data. The median IDR was 0.32 seroconversions per cattle-year at risk with a range from 0 to 3.45. A confidence interval for the median IDR was estimated based on the Wilcoxon signed-rank procedure (Daniel 1978). The 95% confidence interval for median IDR was 0 to 0.54 seroconversions per cattle-year at risk.

Seroconversion seemed to vary spatially (highest risk in the eastern coast of Queensland) and temporally (highest risk between April and July), but these effects were not statistically evaluated.

TIME VALUE OF HISTORIC TESTING INFORMATION

A herd-level Monte Carlo simulation model has been developed to account for the time between testing and the current assessment of the likelihood of disease freedom (Schlosser and Ebel 2001). This concept has important implications, as the risk of introduction of infection into a herd from other sources often increases with time. In the model, the effective contact rate among herds over time was assumed to be non-zero, and probabilities were modeled as triangular or uniform distributions. In the example used in Schlosser and Ebel (2001), the median value of the sampling evidence of 1,000 test-negative herds from 2 years previous was reduced to 89 negative herds today. Hence, the model provides a useful first approach to down-weighting the value of historic data to yield a present-day sample size equivalent.

MONITORING AND SURVEILLANCE DATA

An objective of a MOSS is the continuous collection of health and disease data and their determinants in a given population over a defined period of time. Monitoring excludes any immediate control activities, whereas surveillance is a specific extension of monitoring in which obtained information is used and measures are taken if certain threshold levels related to disease status have been exceeded (Doherr and Audigé 2001; European Commission 2000; Noordhuizen et al. 1997; Office International des Epizooties [OIE] 1998, 2000). For highly contagious diseases such as foot-and-mouth disease (FMD) and classical swine fever (CSF) but also for noncontagious diseases such as bovine spongiform encephalopathy (BSE), that threshold level is one case: each detected case results in a disease control activity such as culling contact animals. In this section, we focus on the analysis of MOSS data and the evaluation of temporal and spatial patterns of disease in herds. Temporal and spatial analytic methods are described in more detail in Chapters 6 and 7, respectively.

Assessment of Temporal Changes in Prevalence (Proportion of Infected Herds and Within-herd Prevalence)

As part of a MOSS, a population of animals, or herds of animals, is constantly monitored for the occurrence of a specific outcome of interest such as clinical disease, macroscopically visible lesions during carcass examination, or other measurable events of interest. If the temporal frequency of those events is recorded, a proportion of individuals examined per unit time that actually were recorded with the events can be calculated. This proportion, depending on the exact definition of the numerator (cases) and the denominator (population at risk of being or becoming a case), can be expressed as a period prevalence, a cumulative incidence, or an incidence rate (or incidence density) for a defined period of time (Thrusfield 1995). The accumulation of a series of such proportions for consecutive time periods will result in a curve depicting the pattern of disease in that population over time. For simplification, however, these so-called epidemic curves often only present the number of new cases (the numerator) per time period rather than the proportion. Examples are the epidemic curve of the recent FMD outbreak in the United Kingdom (Figure 5.2), the number of BSE cases in Switzerland (Figure 5.3), and the number of CSF outbreaks recorded in Europe between 1960 and 1998 (Figure 5.4). Under the assumption that the observed reference population did not change over time and that the system for detecting cases was comparable between time periods, one can expect a similar pattern when reproducing those epidemic curves with prevalence or incidence measures on the *y*-axis rather than with crude case numbers. On the basis of the units of the denominator and its own changes over time, however, the figures for the same disease can vary.

The main objectives of drawing such epidemic curves are to visualize existing temporal trends and to describe the type of outbreak; for example, point source or propagated. It might also be possible to estimate incubation times of propagated epidemics. Epidemic curves are useful during periods of low disease occurrence for making decisions about the need for control measures whenever the disease frequency per unit time exceeds a predefined threshold

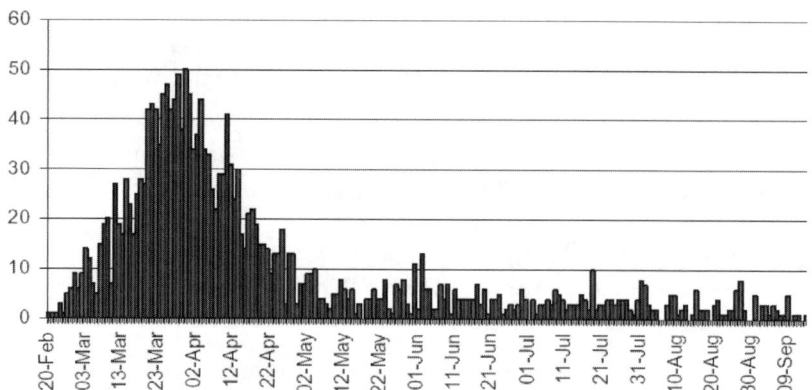

FIGURE 5.2   Epidemic curve for foot-and-mouth disease in the United Kingdom, 2001 (from the DEFRA Web site; http://www.defra.gov.uk).

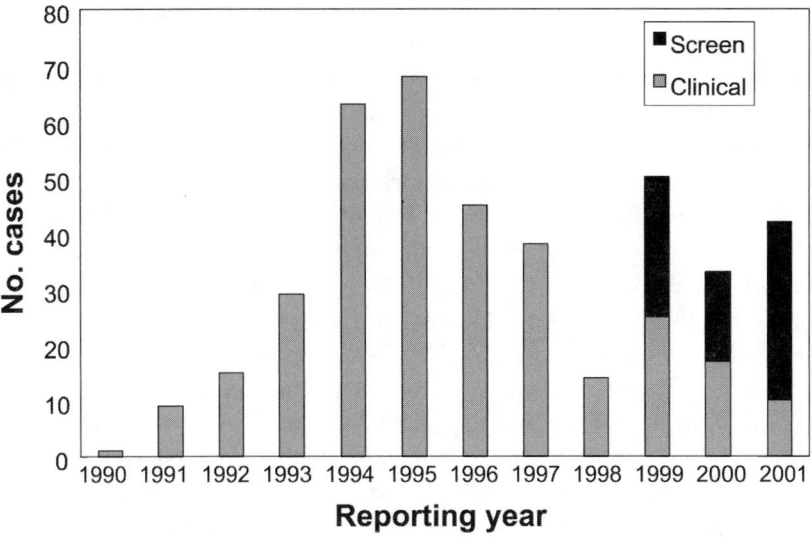

FIGURE 5.3   Annual number of bovine spongiform encephalopathy cases detected clinically or by screening at slaughter in Switzerland between 1990 and 2001 (from the Swiss Federal Veterinary Office; http://www.BVET.ch).

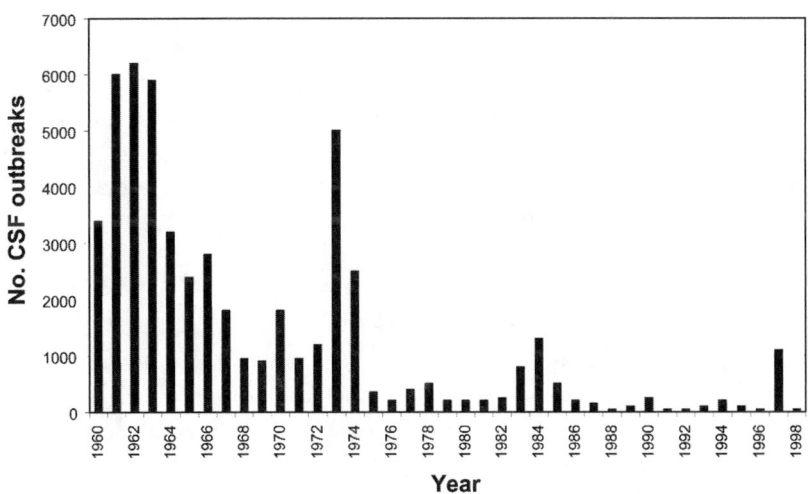

FIGURE 5.4   Classical swine fever cases in Europe between 1960 and 1998 (from European Union statistics; http://www.europa.eu.int/comm/eurostat/Public/datashop/print-catalogue/EN?catalo).

level. During a disease outbreak or disease eradication process, it is important to monitor the reduction in disease frequency as a function of the immediate or delayed effect of the implemented control measures such as culling of infected and exposed herds or the ban on use of ruminant-derived meat-and-bone meal (MBM) in cattle feed (Doherr 2002). The time delay in detecting the effects of control measures is especially pronounced in the example of BSE. The Swiss MBM ban implemented at the end of 1990 resulted in a drop in the number of clinical cases after 1995 (Figure 5.3). This is attributable to the long incubation period of BSE. For other diseases such as FMD, measures such as quarantine or herd depopulation, implemented shortly after case detection, result in a turn of the epidemic within weeks (Figure 5.2).

Another objective of drawing epidemic curves, or evaluating individual time periods, is to compare disease frequency between different populations, often defined by geographic regions such as states or countries. Statistical tests for the comparison of proportions such as the chi-square or Fisher exact tests can be used to assess whether an observed difference in disease frequency between these populations or between different time points within the same population truly exists. An alternative approach to compare such prevalence estimates is the calculation of odds ratios and 95% confidence intervals.

There are a number of situations in which disease frequency estimates per unit time are not comparable either for the same geographic region and different time points or for populations from different geographic regions at the same time point. The main reasons for this lack of comparability are temporal changes or among-population differences in the case detection system, such as new disease definition or the use of different diagnostic tests (numerator), and differences in the size or the definition of the population-at-risk (denominator).

Careful evaluation is needed to determine whether it is justifiable to compare two population proportions derived for different time points or for different populations to draw unbiased conclusions from that comparison.

Modeling of Epidemics in Time and Space Alone or in Combination with Survey Data

For the evaluation of past or current epidemics, modeling has become a standard tool in human and veterinary epidemiology. The initial objective of such models often is to build a simplified structure (the model) that will simulate (reconstruct) a past epidemic in a given population over time with reasonable precision. Past MOSS data are required for the model building process, and the precision of the model results is a direct function of the quality (completeness) of the MOSS data. Alternatively, knowledge of the biologic structure of the population as well as risk factors for diseases can be used to generate such models. Here, MOSS data initially are not required for model building; however, no model can be validated without comparison of the model predictions with real (observed) data. Such data are typically collected during MOSS activities. In both approaches, models subsequently are used for predictions, about the future course of the epidemic, the effectiveness of control scenarios, or the potential exposure of other species. Several such models have been published for BSE (Anderson et al. 1996; Cohen et al. 2000; Doherr et al. 1999; Donnelly et al. 1997, 1999a, 1999b; Ferguson et al. 1997, 1998), the new variant of Creutzfeldt-Jacob disease (CJD; Cohen 2000; Ghani et al. 1998, 2000), and the 2001 FMD outbreak in the United Kingdom (Ferguson et al. 2001; Keeling et al. 2001; Morris et al. 2001). General problems arising from modeling include the lack of information on important parameters in the model (assumptions have to be made) and the unreliability of existing information. In both instances, the model predictions will differ from the observed data, and not only will the validity of the model be questioned, but the value of modeling per se also will be questioned. One of the major values of all models, however, is that it will force the investigators to identify the major contributing factors to and their main interactions with an epidemic. During the model building process, a considerable amount of insight is gained into these risk factors, and areas in which data are missing or unreliable are identified. New hypotheses are generated and areas for future research are defined.

CONCLUSION

In this chapter, analyses of data from surveys conducted at a single time point (prevalence) or from repeated surveys (prevalence and incidence) were considered. Estimation assuming perfect and imperfect tests and disease clustering is described. This chapter emphasized traditional frequentist statistical methods, but an outline of the Bayesian approach to analysis of survey data was also addressed.

BIBLIOGRAPHY

Anderson R.M., Donnelly C.A., Ferguson N.M., Woolhouse M.E., Watt C.J., Udy H.J., MaWhinney S., Dunstan S.P., Southwood T.R., Wilesmith J.W., Ryan J.B., Hoinville L.J., Hillerton J.E., Austin A.R., Wells G.A.H. 1996. Transmission dynamics and epidemiology of BSE in British cattle. Nature 382:779–788.

Audigé L., Beckett S. 1999. A quantitative assessment of the validity of animal health surveys using stochastic modelling. Prev Vet Med 38:277–288.

Audigé L., Doherr M.D., Hauser R., Salman, M.D. 2001. Stochastic modelling as a tool for planning animal-health surveys and interpreting screening-test results. Prev Vet Med 49:1–17.

Blyth, C.R. 1986. Approximate binomial confidence limits. J Am Stat Assoc 81:843–855.

Cameron A.R., Baldock F.C. 1998a. A new probability formula for surveys to substantiate freedom from disease. Prev Vet Med 34:1–17.

Cameron A.R., Baldock F.C. 1998b. Two-stage sampling in surveys to substantiate freedom from disease. Prev Vet Med 34:19–30.

Canon N., Audigé L., Denac H., Hofman M., Griot C. 1998. Evidence of freedom from porcine reproductive and respiratory syndrome (PRRS) virus infection in Switzerland. Vet Rec 142(6):142–143.

Casella G., George E.I. 1992. Explaining the Gibbs sampler. Am Stat 46:167–174.

Christensen J., Gardner I.A. 2000. Herd-level interpretation of diagnostic tests. Prev Vet Med 45:83–106.

Cohen C. 2000. Does improvement in case ascertainment explain the increase in sporadic Creutzfeldt-Jakob disease since 1970 in the United Kingdom? Am J Epidemiol 152(5):474–479.

Cohen C., Heim D., Doherr M.G., Stärk K.D.C. 2000. Age,-cohort models to forecast the BSE epidemic in the United Kingdom and in Switzerland. In: *Proceedings of the Ninth International Society on Veterinary Epidemiology and Economics*, Breckenridge, CO, Abstract #230.

Cowling D.W., Gardner I.A., Johnson W.O. 1999. Comparison of methods for estimation of individual-level prevalence based on pooled samples. Prev Vet Med 39:211–225.

Daniel W.W. 1978. Applied nonparametric statistics, 2nd ed. PWS-Kent, Boston, pp 45–48.

Doherr M.G. 2002. Bovine spongiform encephalopathy (BSE)—Infectious, contagious, zoonotic, or production disease? Acta Vet Scand (in press).

Doherr M.G., Audigé L. 2001. Monitoring and surveillance for rare health-related events—A review from the veterinary perspective. Philos Trans R Soc Lond B Biol Sci 356:1097–1106.

Doherr M.G., Heim D., Vandevelde M., Fatzer R. 1999. Modelling the expected numbers of preclinical and clinical cases of bovine spongiform encephalopathy in Switzerland. Vet Rec 145(6):155–60.

Donald A. 1993. Prevalence estimation using diagnostic tests when there are multiple, correlated disease states in the same animal or farm. Prev Vet Med 15:125–145.

Donald A., Donner A. 1987. Adjustments to the mantel haenszel chi-square statistic and odds ratio variance estimator when the data are clustered. Stat Med 6:491–499.

Donnelly C.A., Ferguson N.M., Ghani A.C., Woolhouse M.E., Watt C.J., Anderson R.M. 1997. The epidemiology of BSE in cattle herds in Great Britain. I. Epidemiological processes, demography of cattle and approaches to control by culling. Philos Trans R Soc Lond B Biol Sci 352(1355):781–801.

Donnelly C.A., Santos R., Ramos M., Galo A., Simas J.P. 1999a. BSE in Portugal: Anticipating the decline of an epidemic. J Epidemiol Biostat 4(4):277–283.

Donnelly C.A., MaWhinney S., Anderson R.M. 1999b. A review of the BSE epidemic in British cattle. Ecosystem Health 5(3):164–173.

Donner A., Donald A. 1987. Analysis of data arising from a stratified design with the cluster as unit of randomization. Stat Med 6:43–52.

European Commission. 2000. Proposal for a Directive of the European Parliament and the Council on the monitoring of zoonoses and agents thereof and repealing Council Directive 92/117/EEC. Working document SANCO/2929/99-Rev. 2, Commission of the European Communities, Brussels, Belgium.

Ferguson N.M., Donnelly C.A., Woolhouse M.E., Anderson R.M. 1997. The epidemiology of BSE in cattle herds in Great Britain. II. Model construction and analysis of transmission dynamics. Philos Trans R Soc Lond B Biol Sci 352(1355):803–838.

Ferguson N.M., Ghani A.C., Donnelly C.A., Denny G.O., Anderson R.M. 1998. BSE in Northern Ireland: Epidemiological patterns past, present and future. Philos Trans R Soc Lond B Biol Sci 265(1396):545–554.

Ferguson N.M., Donnelly C.A., Anderson R.M. 2001. Transmission intensity and impact of control policies on the foot and mouth epidemic in Great Britain. Nature 413:542–548.

Gard G.P., Shorthose J.E., Weir R.P., Walsh S.J., Melville L.F. 1988. Arboviruses recovered from sentinel livestock in northern Australia. Vet Microbiol 18:109–118.

Ghani A.C., Ferguson N.M., Donnelly C.A., Hagenaars, T.J., Anderson R.M. 1998. Epidemiological determinants of the pattern and magnitude of the vCJD epidemic in Great Britain. Philos Trans R Soc Lond B Biol Sci 265(1413):2443–2452.

Ghani A.C., Ferguson N.M., Donnelly C.A., Anderson, R.M. 2000. Predicted vCJD mortality in Great Britain. Nature 406(6796):583–584.

Gohm D.S., Thur B., Audigé L., Hofmann M.A. 1999. A survey of Newcastle disease in Swiss laying-hen flocks using serological testing and simulation modelling. Prev Vet Med 38:277–288.

Greiner M., Gardner I.A. 2000. Application of diagnostic tests in veterinary epidemiologic studies. Prev Vet Med 45:43–60.

Jordan D., McEwen S.A. 1998. Herd-level test performance based on uncertain estimates of individual test performance, individual true prevalence and herd true prevalence. Prev Vet Med 36:187–209.

Keeling M.J., Woolhouse M.E.J., Shaw D.J., Matthews L., Chase-Topping M., Haydon D.T., Cornell S.J., Kappey J., Wilesmith J., Grenfell B.T. 2001. Dynamics of the 2001 UK Foot and Mouth Epidemic: Stochastic dispersal in a heterogeneous landscape. Science 294:813–817.

Martin S.W., Shoukri M., Thorburn M.A. 1992. Evaluating the health status of herds based on tests applied to individuals. Prev Vet Med 75:596–600.

McDermott J.J., Schukken Y.H. 1994. A review of methods used to adjust for cluster effects in explanatory epidemiological studies of animal populations. Prev Vet Med 18:155–173.

Morris R.S., Wilesmith J.W., Stern M.W., Sanson R.L., Stevenson M.A. 2001. Predictive spatial modelling of alternative control strategies for the foot-and-mouth disease epidemic in Great Britain. Vet Rec 149(5):137–44.

Noordhuizen J.P.T.M., Frankena K., van der Hoofd C.M., Graat E.A.M. (Eds.). 1997. Application of quantitative methods in veterinary epidemiology. Wageningen Press, Wageningen, The Netherlands.

Office International des Epizooties. 1998. Guide to epidemiological surveillance for rinderpest. Rev Sci Technique 17(3):796–824.

Office International des Epizooties. 2000. Recommended standard for epidemiological surveillance systems for Rinderpest. Office International des Epizooties, International Animal Health Code Part 3, Section 3.8, Appendix 3.8.1, pp 1–7; http://www.oie.int/.

Ridout M.S., Demetrio C.G.B., Firth D. 1999. Estimating intraclass correlation for binary data. Biometrics 55:137–148.

Robert C.P., Casella G. 1999. Monte Carlo statistical methods. Springer, New York.

Rogan W.J., Gladen B. 1978. Estimating prevalence from the results of a screening test. Am J Epidemiol 107:71–76.

Schlosser W., Ebel E. 2001. Use of a Markov chain Monte Carlo model to evaluate the time value of historical testing information in animal populations. Prev Vet Med 48:167–175.

Sørensen V., Barfod K., Feld N.C. 1992. Evaluation of a monoclonal blocking ELISA and IHA for antibodies to Mycoplasma hyopneumoniae in SPF-pig herds. Vet Rec 130:488–490.

Sørensen V., Barfod K., Feld N.C., Vraa-Andersen L. 1993. Application of enzyme-immunosorbent assay for the surveillance of Mycoplasma hyopneumoniae infection in pigs. Rev Sci Tech des Int Epizoot 12:593–604.

Suess E.A., Gardner I.A., Johnson W.O. 2002. Hierarchical Bayesian model for prevalence inferences and determination of a country's status for an animal disease. Prev Vet Med 55:155–171.

Thrusfield M. 1995. Describing disease occurrence. In: Veterinary epidemiology, 2nd ed. Blackwell Science, Oxford, pp 37–56.

United States Department of Agriculture. 1997. Johne's disease on U.S. dairy operations. USDA:APHIS:VS, CEAH, National Animal Health Monitoring System. Fort Collins, CO #N245.1097.

Vose D. 1996. Quantitative risk analysis—a guide to Monte Carlo simulation modelling. Wiley, Chichester.

Ward M.P., Flanagan M., Carpenter T.E., Hird D.W., Thurmond M.C., Johnson S.J., Dashorst M.E. 1995. Infection of cattle with bluetongue viruses in Queensland, Australia: Results of a sentinel herd study, 1990–1992. Vet Microbiol 45:35–44.

Wells S.J., Wagner B.A. 2000. Herd-level risk factors for infection with *Mycobacterium paratuberculosis* in US dairies and association between familiarity of the herd manager with the disease or prior diagnosis of the disease in that herd and use of preventive measures. J Am Vet Med Assoc 216:1450–1457.

Methods for Determining Temporal Clusters in Surveillance and Survey Programs

T.E. Carpenter[1] and M.P. Ward[2]

INTRODUCTION

Disease surveillance and survey programs enable veterinarians and others involved with the well being of animals to detect either the emergence of a new disease or an unusual increase (epidemic) in an endemic disease. Deciding whether or not disease events are clustered may be obvious in some cases, and simply plotting the time-series of events will reveal clustering. However, in other cases, the temporal clustering may be subtle. In addition, describing and comparing two or more disease patterns may be difficult based simply on the

[1]Department of Medicine and Epidemiology, School of Veterinary Medicine, University of California, Davis, CA 95616
[2]Department of Veterinary Pathobiology, School of Veterinary Medicine, Purdue University, West Lafayette, IN 47907–2027

visual interpretation of plotted time-series. In these situations, statistical techniques may be helpful by introducing objectivity and precision to visual descriptions (Ward and Carpenter 2000b).

Several techniques are available to analyze time-series data generated by surveillance or survey programs. Time-series analysis is a technique, applied in specific research situations in veterinary medicine, to describe or predict the temporal distribution of diseases (Cherry et al. 1998; Courtin et al. 2000; Curk and Carpenter 1994; Doherr et al. 1999; Ekstrand and Carpenter 1998; French et al. 1999; Nrgaard et al 1999; Ward 2002; Ward and Johnson 1996). Although useful in describing long-term and cyclical patterns and identifying unusual deviations, time-series analysis requires a relatively long series of observations, typically well in excess of 50, and is thus inappropriate for many relatively new health surveillance or survey situations.

Besides time-series analysis, at least seven other statistical techniques have been developed or adopted for use in health surveillance systems. These techniques are designed to detect, both rapidly and efficiently, unusual increases in morbidity or mortality. These are the matrix (Jacquez 1994), Poisson (Christensen and Rudemo 1996, 1998; Flynt 1974), negative binomial (Hill et al. 1968; Weatherall and Haskey 1976), two-stage (Hardy et al. 1990), sets (Chen 1986, 1987; Chen et al. 1982), scan (Naus 1982; Wallenstein 1980; Wallenstein and Neff 1987), and cusum (Bjerkdal and Bakketeig 1975; Ewan and Kemp 1960; Healy 1968; Kennett and Pollack 1983) techniques. In this chapter, the scan technique will be presented to illustrate the application of a temporal cluster test to identify an increase in morbidity or mortality.

Analysis of the temporal distribution of health events can have four aims: rapid identification of clusters of events, identification of confounders and risk factors for clusters, generation or confirmation of a research hypothesis, and confirmation of the etiology of a disease process that has been observed (Carpenter 2001; Ward and Carpenter 2000a).

The rapid development of disease surveillance and monitoring systems, herd health programs, and geographical information systems in the last three decades has enabled veterinary epidemiologists to routinely test hypotheses regarding disease causation and a large number of putative causal factors. However, an important step to take before searching for causes of disease is to determine whether disease occurrence is clustered. If disease occurrence is not temporally clustered, then causal hypothesis testing may be futile (Ward and Carpenter 2000a). The purpose of this chapter is to present and illustrate a commonly used statistical test (specifically, the scan test) that may be used for the detection of increased number of adverse health events occurring in a time-series survey.

SCAN TEST

The scan statistic test (Naus 1965; Wallenstein 1980; Weinstock 1981) is used to detect temporal clustering of events in a defined population. Although the test focuses on occurrences of an event, for example, cases of disease, it presumes that the size of the population at risk of the disease of interest is relatively constant over the study period. The scan test evaluates a time-series of events using intervals (windows) to determine the maximum number of events that occur within each fixed window, or time period.

First, we will assume that the total number of cases occurring in the population (N) is known. The question is what is the probability of observing number (n) of cases in a time period (such as month) when N cases were reported over the T-month study period? The equation is

$$P = Pr(n, N, r), \tag{1}$$

where $r = w/T$ and w is the width of the time window selected.

The formulation of the calculations needed to determine P was derived by Wallenstein and Neff (1987):

$$P = Pr(n, N, r) = (n/r - N + 1) \times Pr(M = n) + 2Pr[M \geq (n + 1)], \tag{2}$$

where M has a binomial distribution with parameters N and $p = r$. Note that this equation gives the exact probability, as derived by Naus (1965), when $n > N/2$ and $r < 0.5$ and is meant as a good approximation otherwise. Continuing,

$$Pr(M = n) = \frac{N!}{(N - n)!n!} r^n (1 - r)^{N-n}, \tag{3}$$

where the initial factorial-term can be rewritten as a combinatory process for calculation purposes (e.g., EXCEL [Microsoft, Redmond, WA] cannot perform factorial calculations for $N > 170$, whereas combinatorial values may be calculated with $N > 100,000$, using the same program):

$$\frac{N!}{(N - n)!n!} = \binom{N}{n}, \tag{4}$$

and M is the maximum number of cases observed in a window. The calculated value of P is compared with the predefined type-I error (usually 0.05) to determine whether the number of adverse health events may be explained by chance only (i.e., the random error).

CASE STUDIES

SALMONELLA IN CALIFORNIA

To illustrate this test, we will use data collected from two studies designed to better understand the time-space distribution of *Salmonella* infections in livestock examined either at a diagnostic laboratory system or a school of veterinary medicine teaching hospital.

In the first study, 57 *Salmonella* Montevideo isolates were obtained from adult diarrheic cattle in California and submitted to the California Animal Health and Food Safety Laboratory System (CAHFS) during a 90-month period (February 1991 through June 1998). The temporal distribution of *S.* Montevideo isolates obtained in this study is shown in Figure 6.1.

The maximum number of isolates ($n = 5$) obtained in a single month occurred in October 1996. Using eq. (1), the probability of obtaining exactly five isolates in a single month is calculated as

$$Pr(M = 5) = \frac{57!}{(57 - 5)!5!}(1/90)^5[1 - (1/90)]^{57-5}. \tag{5}$$

The probability of observing this number may be calculated by entering the above equation into a spreadsheet program or using a spreadsheet-resident equation. For example, this is accomplished in EXCEL by double-clicking the f_x

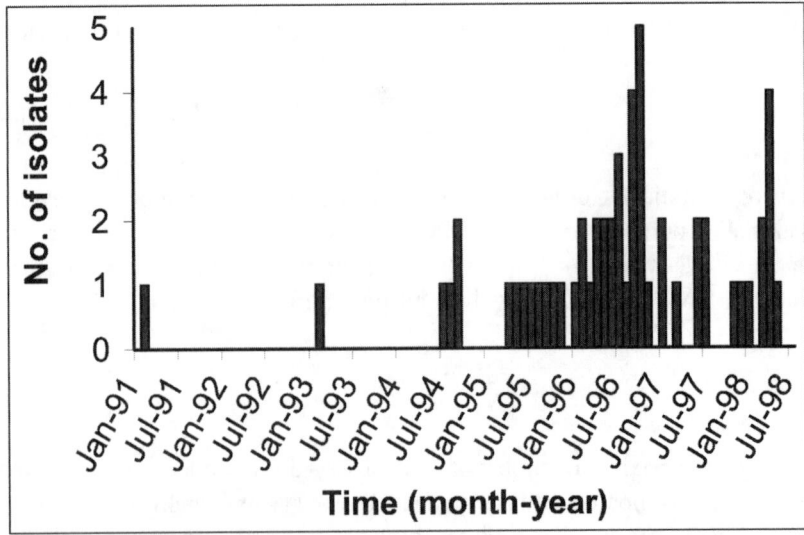

FIGURE 6.1   Temporal distribution of *Salmonella* Montevideo isolates obtained from adult diarrheic dairy cattle in California, February 1991 through June 1998.

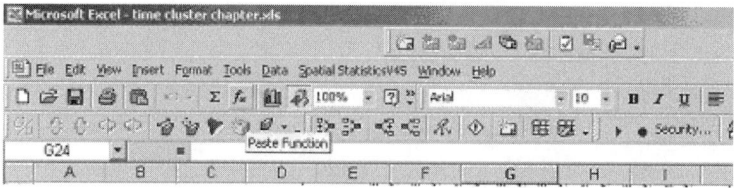

FIGURE 6.2   Illustration of "Paste Function" feature available in a computer spreadsheet.

button ("Paste Function"), located between the S; and chart buttons, in the standard toolbar (third) row in the menu bar at the top of the spreadsheet (see Figure 6.2).

This action will activate the function category box (Figure 6.3), from which the binomial distribution may be calculated by selecting BINOMDIST from the "Function name" window.

Once selected, the user inputs values for n (Number_s), N (Trial_s), r (Probability_s), and whether the function calculates a probability density function (pdf) or cumulative distribution function (CDF; cumulative $= 0$ or 1 for a pdf or CDF, respectively; see Figure 6.4).

Hence, the probability of observing exactly five cases in a single month is calculated as

$$Pr(M = 5) = 0.000397.$$

The next step in calculating the scan test probability is to determine the probability of observing at least one more than the observed n, $Pr[M \geq (n + 1)]$. The

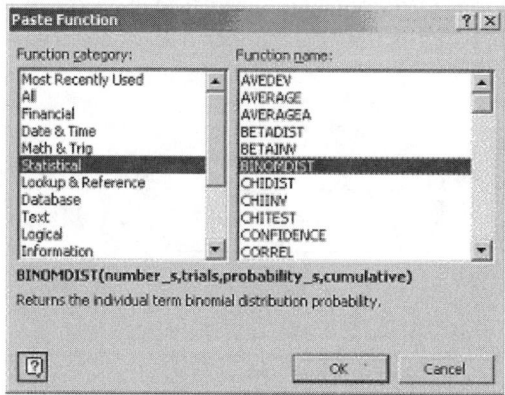

FIGURE 6.3   Illustration of the binomial equation as one of several functions available in a spreadsheet program.

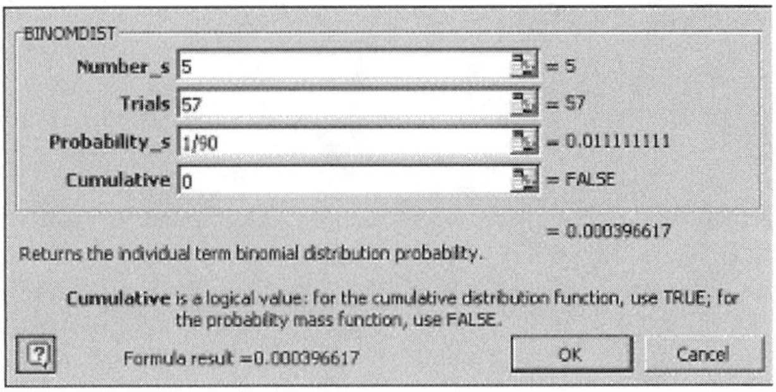

FIGURE 6.4   Illustration of spreadsheet menu for creating a binomial probability density function (pdf).

calculation may be simplified by calculating the probability of not observing n or fewer cases, because this would entail a potentially large number of calculations ($n + 1$ through $n + N$). This approach simplifies to the calculation of the CDF of n cases (see Figure 6.5) and then subtracting this value from 1.

The cumulative probability of observing 0 to 5 is calculated as the sum of the probability density functions for $P(X = 0, 1, \ldots 5)$, and is 0.99995790. The probability of observing ≥ 6 may be calculated as $Pr(M \geq 6) = 1 - 0.99995790 = 0.0000420$.

Using these calculations, the probability of observing a cluster of five cases in one month, where a total of 57 isolates were obtained in 90 months, is calculated as $P = Pr(5, 57, 1/90) = [5/(1/90) - 57 + 1] \times 0.000397 + 2 \times 0.0000420 = 0.1565$.

The conclusion is that it is not ($P = .16$) statistically significant to obtain five isolates of *S.* Montevideo from adult diarrheic dairy cattle in 1 month during the study period, based on the total number of *S.* Montevideo obtained during

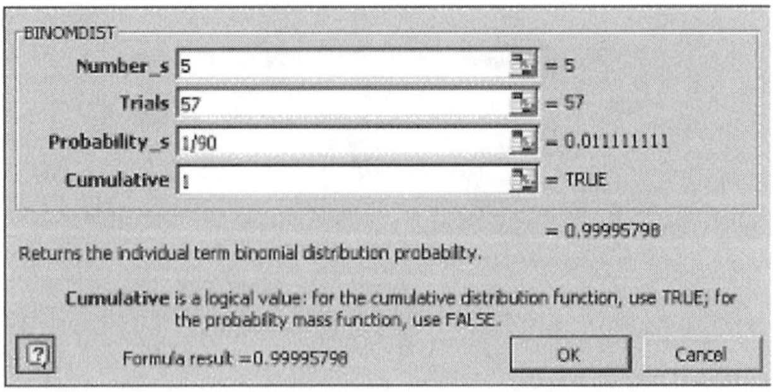

FIGURE 6.5   Illustration of spreadsheet menu for creating a binomial cumulative distribution function (CDF).

the study. In addition to examining the statistical significance of the number of events occurring in a single time period, it is often of interest to examine multiple consecutive time periods to identify possible disease etiologies. In the case of the S. Montevideo survey, the maximum number of this serotype in a specified consecutive time period was examined for window widths (w) corresponding to 2 to 8 consecutive months. This examination indicated a consistent pattern; that is the maximum number of cases in consecutive months occurred at and before October 1996 (Table 6.1). The statistical significance of these observations is tested similarly, as described earlier. To illustrate, we will calculate the significance of obtaining nine S. Montevideo isolates during September and October 1996.

Thus, the probability of observing 9 cases in 2 consecutive months is calculated as

$$Pr(M = 9) = \frac{57!}{(57 - 9)!9!}(2/90)^9[(1 - (2/90)]^{57-9} = 0.00000404284 \quad (6)$$

Continuing, we calculate the probability of not obtaining 10 or more isolates in 2 consecutive months as the probability of not obtaining nine or fewer isolates, as $Pr(M \geq 10) = 1 - Pr(M \leq 9)$, where it should be noted the probability changes from 1/90 to 2/90, and $Pr(M \leq 9) = 0.999999512$ and $Pr(M \geq 10) = 1 - 0.999999512 = 0.000000487913$.

TABLE 6.1   Number (Using Windows of 1–8 Months) of *Salmonella* Montevideo Isolates Obtained from Adult Diarrheic Dairy Cattle in California, March 1996 through February 1997

Date	Window width (months)							
	1	2	3	4	5	6	7	8
1996								
March	1	3	4	4	5	6	7	8
April	2	3	5	6	6	7	8	9
May	2	4	5	7	8	8	9	10
June	2	4	6	7	9	10	10	11
July	3	5	7	9	10	12	13	13
August	1	4	6	8	10	11	13	14
September	4	5	8	10	12	14	15	17
October	5	**9**	**10**	**13**	**15**	**17**	**19**	**20**
November	1	6	**10**	11	14	16	18	**20**
December	0	1	6	10	11	14	16	18
1997								
January	2	2	3	8	12	13	16	18
February	0	2	2	3	8	12	13	16

Note. Window-maxima are in bold.

Using these calculations, the probability of observing a cluster of nine cases in 2 consecutive months, where a total of 57 isolates were obtained in 90 months, is calculated as $P = Pr(9, 57, 2/90) = [9/(2/90) - 57 + 1] \times 0.00000404284 + 2 \times 0.000000487913 = 0.00141$.

Thus, it may be concluded that it was statistically significant ($P = .001$) that nine isolates were obtained during September and October 1996. Similarly significant temporal clustering was observed for up to 8 consecutive months (Table 6.2).

The temporal clustering of S. Montevideo isolates obtained over the 90-month survey period, in which the total number of isolates obtained was 57, is shown in Figure 6.1. Visually, it can be seen that the first isolate was obtained in February 1991, and until July 1994, only one more isolate was obtained. A consistent pattern of about one isolate per month occurred between April 1995 and January 1996. The maximum monthly number of isolates (five) was obtained in October 1996. The scan test identified significant clusters occurring in window widths of 2 to 8 months, from March through October 1996. The presence of such a multiple-month time cluster supports the argument that these epidemics were the result of interfarm transmission and not caused by point-source infections alone, which would tend to occur as shorter, for example, single month, epidemics. Temporal clusters such as the one observed with S. Montevideo isolates imply a more sporadic, endemic occurrence.

SALMONELLA IN INDIANA

In the second study, a total of 494 horses were admitted to a veterinary teaching hospital in Indiana between October 2000 and June 2001. At least three fecal samples were collected and cultured for *Salmonella* species from 232 of these horses. None of the 232 horses included in the study was diagnosed with clinical salmonellosis. Only four horses in the survey were admitted with a presenting complaint of diarrhea, and none of these horses presented with fever.

Salmonella was isolated from 12 of the 232 horses, with S. Newport C2 being the most prevalent serotype. The temporal distribution of *Salmonella* isolations is shown in Figure 6.6. No statistically significant clustering was found when the temporal distribution of cases over a period of 1 to 14 days was examined using the scan test ($.77 \leq P \leq 1.00$). For illustrative purposes, we further examined potential clusters on a weekly basis, from 14 to 28 days each. The results were again not statistically significant ($.18 \leq P \leq .43$; Table 6.3). Although no statistically significant temporal clusters of *Salmonella* isolations were observed, two clusters were noteworthy. The first was a cluster of five cases occurring within a 28-day period (November 4 through December 1, 2000; weeks 5 to 8). The second involved a smaller cluster of three cases ap-

TABLE 6.2 Scan Test Results for the Detection of Temporal Clustering of 57 *Salmonella* Montevideo Isolates Obtained from Adult Diarrheic Dairy Cattle in California during a 90-Month period, February 1991 through June 1998

	Window width (w = months)							
	1	2	3	4	5	6	7	8
Maximum cases (M)	5	9	10	13	15	17	19	20
Time period ($r = w$/total months)	0.01111	0.02222	0.03333	0.04444	0.05556	0.06667	0.07778	0.08889
$P(M = n)$	.000397	.000004	.00001	.0000009	.0000003	.00000009	.00000002	.00000004
$P(M \geq n+1)$	.00004	.0000005	.000003	.0000001	.00000005	.00000002	.00000005	.000000007
$P(n, N, r)$	.15635	.00141	.00363	.00021	.00006	.00002	.000005	.000006

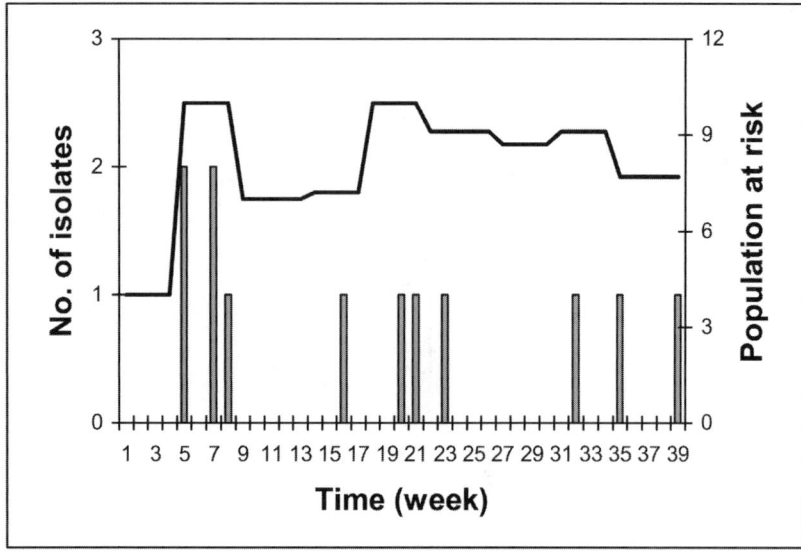

FIGURE 6.6   Temporal distribution of 12 *Salmonella* isolates (bars) obtained from horses admitted to an Indiana hospital, October 14, 2000 (week 1), through June 30, 2001 (week 39). The average daily population of horses at-risk, for each study month, is shown (line).

TABLE 6.3   Scan Test Results for the Detection of Temporal Clustering of 12 Cases of *Salmonella* Isolates Obtained from Horses in an Indiana Hospital during a 260-Day Period, October 14, 2000, through June 30, 2001

	Window width		
Window width (w = days)	14	21	28
Maximum cases (M)	3	4	5
Time period ($r = w$/total days)	0.053846	0.080769	0.107692
$P(M = n)$	.020871	.01074	.005167
$P(M \geq n + 1)$	.002933	.001677	.000809
$P(n, N, r)$	.939096	.417082	.184682

pearing over a 21-day period (February 24 through March 16, 2001; weeks 21 to 23). The average population of horses at risk of *Salmonella* shedding during the survey is also shown in Figure 6.6. Although the population fluctuated during the period, it remained within a range of approximately 7 to 10 horses per day. No significant ($P = .26$) linear trend in the population at risk during the study period was detected. Therefore, the assumption of an approximately constant population at risk during the study period is probably met in this example. The only exception was during the first few weeks of the survey, in which there were only on average approximately four horses at risk per day. This can probably be examined by the phase-in operational period of the survey.

During the period of this survey, 24 isolates were obtained from the 12 horses. *Salmonella* was isolated on one, two, three, or four occasions from five, three, three, and one horse, respectively. The following *Salmonella* serotypes (number) were isolated: *S.* Thompson C1 (three), *S.* Typhimurium B (four), *S.* Newport C2 (nine), *S.* Reading B (three), *S.* Hartford C1 (two), *S.* Java B (two), and *S.* Senftenberg E4 (one). These isolates were recovered from fecal samples from one, three, four, one, one, two, and one horse, respectively. One horse was apparently coinfected with *S.* Typhimurium and *S.* Newport; only one specific serotype was recovered from the other 11 horses. The temporal distribution of isolation of serotypes is shown in Table 6.4. Serotype-specific clustering, using a window of length of up to 28 days, was examined for serotypes *S.* Typhimurium B, *S.* Newport C2, and *S.* Java B. No clustering was detected (*S.* Typhimurium B, $.68 \leq P \leq .82$; *S.* Newport C2, $.77 \leq P \leq .78$; and *S.* Java B, $.24 \leq P \leq .45$).

Results from this analysis indicate that isolates of *Salmonella* obtained from the study population were not temporally clustered. On the basis of this information, it can be concluded that there was no evidence of nosocomial transmission of *Salmonella* within the hospital during the study period.

PRECAUTIONS

It should be noted that this test and other temporal-cluster tests are sensitive and potentially biased because of population at-risk dynamics. Specifically, it

TABLE 6.4   *Salmonella* Species Isolates Obtained from Horses in an Indiana Hospital during a 260-Day Period, October 14, 2000, through June 30, 2001

Horse number	Serotype	Week*
1	Newport C2	5
2	Typhimurium B	5
3	Thompson C1	7
4	Newport C2, Typhimurium B	7
5	Hartford C	8
6	Newport C2	16
7	Typhimurium B	20
8	Newport C2	21
9	Senftenberg E4	23
10	Reading B	32
11	Java B	35
12	Java B	39

*See Figure 5.6.

assumes the population at risk is relatively constant. If, for example, a population were continuously increasing, a bias would be introduced toward clustering of events occurring later in the study period if the number of events occurring was proportional to the size of the population at risk. If the population at risk decreases through the study period, for example, in the case of an infectious disease that either results in mortality or immunity in infected animals, and similarly, if the number of events occurring is proportional to the size of the population at risk, a bias would be introduced toward clustering of events occurring early in the study period. Similarly, recognition and reporting bias should be ruled out as possible explanations for temporal clustering.

CONCLUSIONS

In conclusion, detection of a temporal cluster of events such as disease or illness is one of many steps that may better illuminate the dynamics of a condition. In addition, other statistical tests, including traditional statistical tests such as regression, may be used independently or in combination with temporal, spatial, and temporal-spatial tests to improve the understanding of complex systems associated with these events. A better understanding and more frequent application of these tools should help epidemiologists and others involved with disease control to do their jobs.

BIBLIOGRAPHY

Bjerkdal T., Bakketeig L.S. 1975. Surveillance of congenital malformations and other conditions of the newborn. Int J Epidemiol 4:31–36.

Carpenter T.E. 2001. Methods to investigate spatial and temporal clustering in veterinary epidemiology. Prev Vet Med 48:303–320.

Chen R. 1986. Revised values for the parameters of the sets techniques for monitoring the incidence rate of a rare disease. Methods Inform Med 25:47–49.

Chen R. 1987. The relative efficiency of the sets and the cusum techniques in monitoring the occurrence of a rare event. Stat Med 6:517–525.

Chen R., Mantel N., Connelly R.R., Isacson P. 1982. A monitoring system for chronic diseases. Methods Inform Med 21:86–90.

Cherry B.R., Reeves M.J., Smith G. 1998. Evaluation of bovine viral diarrhea virus control using a mathematical model of infection dynamics. Prev Vet Med 33:91–108.

Christensen J., Rudemo M. 1996. Multiple change-point analysis of disease incidence rates. Prev Vet Med 26:53–76.

Christensen J., Rudemo M. 1998. Multiple change-point analysis applied to the monitoring of salmonella prevalence in Danish pigs and pork. Prev Vet Med 36:131–143.

Courtin F., Carpenter T.E., Paskin R.D., Chomel B.B. 2000. Temporal patterns of domestic and wildlife rabies in Central Namibia stock ranging area, 1986–1996. Prev Vet Med 43:13–28.

Curk A., Carpenter T.E. 1994. Efficacy of the first oral vaccination against fox rabies in Slovenia. Rev Sci Technique 13:763–775.

Doherr M.G., Carpenter T.E., Wilson W.D., Gardner I.A. 1999. Evaluation of temporal and spatial clustering of horses with *Corynebacterium pseudotuberculosis* infection in horses. Am J Vet Res 60:284–291.

Ekstrand C., Carpenter T.E. 1998. Temporal aspects of foot-pad dermatitis in Swedish broilers. Acta Vet Scand 39:229–236.

Ewan W.D., Kemp K.W. 1960. Sampling inspection of continuous processes with no autocorrelation between successive results. Biometrika 47:363–380.

Flynt J.W. 1974. Trends in surveillance of congenital malformations. In: Congenital defects: new directions in research, Janerich A., et al. (Eds.). Academic Press, New York, pp 119–128.

French N.P., Berriatua E., Wall R., Smith K., Morgan K.L. 1999. Sheep scab outbreaks in Great Britain between 1973 and 1992: Spatial and temporal patterns. Vet Parasitol 83:187–200.

Hardy R.J., Schroder G.D., Cooper S.P., Buffler P.A., Prichard H.M., Crane M. 1990. A surveillance system for assessing health effects from hazardous exposures. Am J Epidemiol 132(suppl.):S32-S42.

Healy M.J.R. 1968. The disciplining of medical data. Br Med J 24:210–214.

Hill G.B., Spicer C.C., Weatherall J.A.C. 1968. The computer surveillance of congenital malformations. Br Med Bull 24:215–217.

Jacquez G.M. 1994. Guidelines and procedures for investigating disease clusters. Proceedings of a short course, University of British Columbia. BioMedware, Ann Arbor MI.

Kennett R., Pollack M. 1983. On sequential detection of a shift in the probability of a rare event. J Am Stat Assoc 78:389–395.

Naus J.I. 1965. The distribution of the size of the maximum cluster of points on a line. J Am Stat Assoc 60:532–538.

Naus J.I. 1982. Approximation for distributions of scan statistics. J Am Stat Assoc 77:177–183.

Nrgaard N.H., Lind K.M., Agger J.F. 1999. Cointegration analysis used in a study of dairy-cow mortality. Prev Vet Med 42:99–119.

Wallenstein S. 1980. A test for detection of clustering over time. Am J Epidemiol 111:367–371.

Wallenstein S., Neff N. 1987. An approximation for the distribution of the scan statistic. Stat Med 6:197–207.

Ward M.P. 2002. Seasonality of canine leptospirosis in the United States and Canada and its association with rainfall. Prev Vet Med 56:203–213.

Ward M.P., Carpenter T.E. 2000a. Analysis of time-space clustering in veterinary epidemiology. Prev Vet Med 43:225–237.

Ward M.P., Carpenter T.E. 2000b. Techniques for analysing the clustering of disease in space and in time in veterinary epidemiology. Prev Vet Med 45:257–284.

Ward M.P., Johnson S.J. 1996. Bluetongue virus and the southern oscillation index: Evidence of an association. Prev Vet Med 28:57–68.

Weatherall J.A.C., Haskey J.C. 1976. Surveillance of malformations. Br Med Bull 32:39–44.

Weinstock M.A. 1981. A generalized scan statistic test for the detection of clusters. Am J Epidemiol 10:289–293.

Chapter 7

Methods for Determining Spatial Clusters in Surveillance and Survey Programs

T.E. Carpenter[1] and M.P. Ward[2]

INTRODUCTION

As discussed in Chapter 6, identification of diseases or ill health may be facilitated using a variety of temporal clustering techniques. However, in some situations the disease epidemic may not have a substantial temporal component. In these situations, the epidemic may not be recognized via temporal cluster tests and will be more easily detected by its spatial rather than temporal clustering. With the recent availability of affordable mapping, or geographical information system (GIS), software, identification of spatial clusters has been facilitated. As with cluster analysis of purely time-series data, analysis of the spatial

[1]Department of Medicine and Epidemiology, School of Veterinary Medicine, University of California, Davis, CA 95616

[2]Department of Veterinary Pathobiology, School of Veterinary Medicine, Purdue University, West Lafayette, IN 47907–2027

distribution of health events can have four aims: rapid identification of clusters of events, identification of confounders and risk factors for clusters, generation or confirmation of a research hypothesis, and confirmation of the etiology of a disease process that has been observed (Carpenter 2001; Ward and Carpenter 2000a). Although limited surveillance programs employ statistical techniques to detect temporal clusters of events (see Chapter 6), the same does not appear to be true for the detection of analogous spatial clusters. Traditionally, spatial analysis is limited to describing spatial distributions by mapping the occurrence of the event and visual interpretation.

The study of disease clusters has been relatively common in human epidemiologic research in recent years. Whereas many of the techniques for cluster identification were developed in the 1960s and 1970s, their widespread application and acceptance really did not occur until the 1990s. Several books have been published on the topic of quantifying the spatial statistics and clustering of diseases in populations. Among these, the amount of text devoted to spatial statistics to cluster analysis ranges from a portion of a chapter in a statistical medical research text (Armitage and Berry 1994), a single chapter in an epidemiology text (Selvin 1996), and several textbooks (Alexander and Boyle 1996; Cliff and Ord 1981; Davis 1986; Earickson and Harlin 1994; Ebdon 1985; Elliot et al. 1992; Haining 1990; Krebs 1999; Lawson 2001; McGlashan 1972; Ripley 1988; Thomas 1990; Upton and Fingleton 1985). However, none of these discusses the application of clustering techniques to veterinary problems, which by the nature of the livestock production process, for example, limited life span and movement, or herd characteristics create new problems as well as opportunities for the veterinary epidemiologist in spatial and temporal research.

The rapid development of disease surveillance and monitoring systems, herd health programs, and geographical information systems in the last three decades has enabled veterinary epidemiologists to routinely test hypotheses regarding disease causation and a large number of putative causal factors. However, an important step to take before searching for causes of disease is to determine whether disease occurrence is clustered. If disease occurrence is not spatially clustered, then causal hypothesis testing may be futile (Ward and Carpenter 2000a). The purpose of this chapter is to present and illustrate two commonly used statistical tests (specifically the nearest neighbor and Cuzick-Edwards' tests), which may be used for the detection of increased number of adverse health events detected by a survey or surveillance program in which spatial information is collected.

Numerous cluster analysis techniques have been developed for various types of data, including continuous, dichotomous, rank, and nominal data, as well as various dimensions, including, point, line or transect, and area dimensions

(Carpenter 2001; Moore and Carpenter 1999; Ward and Carpenter 2000b). Although data sometimes may be collected or are summarized on an aggregated level, for example, regional and rank, the precision and power of statistical tests and, consequently, results and interpretations from surveys and surveillance programs are enhanced if the data were analyzed in a less aggregated format; for example, point and count. In this chapter we will illustrate the value of statistical techniques in a survey or surveillance program, focusing on the distribution of point data.

CLUSTER TESTS FOR POINT DATA

The distribution of spatial point data may be random, uniform, or clustered (Figure 7.1). Randomly distributed points, as the name implies, are the distribution one would expect if there were no specific process underlying their distribution. Uniformly distributed points are more regularly or evenly spaced than random points, implying an underlying process of repulsion, as might be expected for wildlife that may be territorial in nature. Clustered points appear

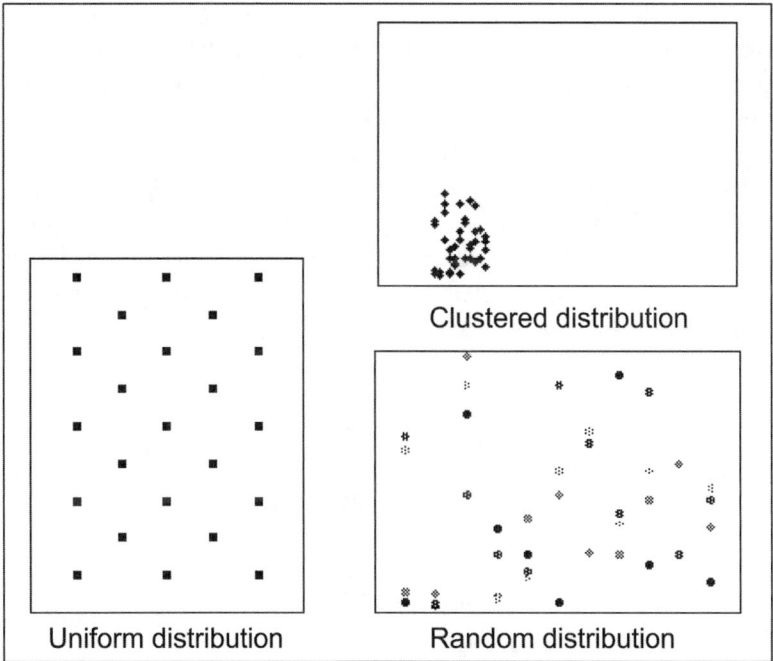

FIGURE 7.1   Examples of alternative point distributions.

more closely together than expected, such as when there is a point source or infectious disease epidemic. In a medical surveillance system, we are typically interested in identifying clusters of disease, as if disease occurs, we expect several spatially clustered cases also to occur because of the process of contagion. Several tests developed to identify spatial clustering of points have been recently reported in the literature (Carpenter 2001; Jacquez et al. 1996a, 1996b; Moore and Carpenter 1999).

In this chapter, we will illustrate methods to detect spatial clusters, using two tests: the nearest neighbor (Clark and Evans 1954) and the Cuzick-Edwards' test (Cuzick and Edwards 1990) on two separate epidemiologic data sets. In both examples, we will first evaluate the level of clustering of case, or outbreak, data; extend the analysis to examine higher levels of clustering; and finally consider the effect of the distribution of the underlying population at risk.

NEAREST NEIGHBOR TECHNIQUE

The most commonly used technique to describe the distribution of point data is the nearest neighbor technique. The nearest neighbor technique measures the mean distance separating closest points (nearest neighbors) and compares these observed values with those expected if the points were randomly distributed. This technique was developed by plant ecologists (Clark and Evans 1954) to evaluate the distribution of arrangements in two and three dimensions, using the nearest neighbor index (R). The index may be used to define individual distributions or to compare two or more spatial distributions. The index ranges from 0 to 2.15, with distributions having a value approximately 0 being closely clustered, those approximately 1 being random, and those approximately 2.15 being uniformly (maximally) distributed or highly dispersed. The index is calculated by dividing the mean distance between nearest neighbor points in a given area ($\overline{D}_{obs}$) by the expected mean distance of a randomly distributed series of points in that area ($\overline{D}_{ran}$) as

$$R = \frac{\overline{D}_{obs}}{\overline{D}_{ran}}. \tag{1}$$

The mean observed distance ($\overline{D}_{obs}$) is calculated by measuring the distance between each nearest neighbor pair and dividing the sum of these distances by the number of points (N), as

$$(\overline{D}_{obs}) = \frac{\sum (d_{ij})}{N}, \tag{2}$$

where d_{ij} is the distance between nearest neighbors i and j. (Note that points i and j may or may not be each other's nearest neighbor; i.e., reflexive pairs.)

The expected mean distance $(\overline{D}_{ran})$ is calculated as

$$\overline{D}_{ran} = \frac{1}{2\sqrt{N/A}} = 0.5\sqrt{A/N}, \tag{3}$$

where A is the size of the study area and N/A is the density of points. By substitution, the index may now be calculated as

$$R = 2(\overline{D}_{obs})\sqrt{\frac{N}{A}}. \tag{4}$$

For example, if $\overline{D}_{obs} = 1$, $N = 20$, and $A = 100$,

$$R = 2(1)\sqrt{\frac{20}{100}} = 0.89, \tag{a}$$

which indicates a random distribution (as the mean observed distance was 1 and a mean distance of 1.1 was expected). The significance of this distribution being nonrandom (i.e., clustered in this case because $0 < R < 1$) may be determined by using the standard deviation of the mean nearest neighbor distance $(\sigma \overline{D}_{ran})$ and calculation of a Z score as

$$\sigma \overline{D}_{ran} = \frac{0.26136}{\sqrt{N(N/A)}}. \tag{5}$$

Therefore,

$$\sigma \overline{D}_{ran} = \frac{0.26136}{\sqrt{20 \times 0.2}} = 0.131. \tag{b}$$

The Z statistic is calculated as

$$z = \frac{\overline{D}_{obs} - \overline{D}_{ran}}{\sigma \overline{D}_{ran}}. \tag{6}$$

In the example,

$$z = \frac{1 - 1.118}{0.131} = -0.90. \tag{c}$$

Positive Z values (i.e., $\overline{D}_{obs} > \overline{D}_{ran}$) denote a more dispersed (uniform) distribution, whereas negative values $(\overline{D}_{ran} > \overline{D}_{obs})$ denote a more clustered distribution, and zero denotes a random distribution. Using a standard table of probabilities associated with Z values for a normal distribution, it may be found that -0.90 corresponds to a probability value of $p = .37$ and that, therefore, the null hypothesis that these points are randomly distributed may not be rejected.

The nearest neighbor analysis discussed above was used to test for the pairwise clustering of points. Therefore, results of statistical tests for the overall point distribution should be interpreted with caution. For example, consider the situation in which pairs of points are very closely associated, as with the classic ballroom dancing example; however, the distribution of all pairs of points are close to uniformly distributed (see Figure 7.2). Using the nearest neighbor test, the conclusion would be that the null hypothesis should be rejected in favor of the alternative hypothesis that the points are clustered. Although this is statistically correct, the conclusions drawn concerning the overall population distribution would be different, emphasizing the importance of correct epidemiologic interpretation of statistical results. A veterinary example illustrating this issue may be testing for clustering of disease in an intensively managed livestock operation. For example, enzootic pneumonia may be highly clustered within pens of finisher pigs, but pens within a shed are uniformly distributed.

Until now, we have examined points being distributed in an area as if they were completely isolated from all influences (points) present in bordering locations. For example, a state or province may examine health data for its population, while (e.g., due to lack of access to necessary data) completely ignoring the association or influence of a neighboring state or province. Therefore, problems may arise from the use of nearest neighbor analysis if the following occurs: the pattern of the data is the result of more than a single process or the data are affected by some unaccounted for boundary data (edge effects). Each of these problems may be taken into account, the former by analyzing higher-order neighbor distances, the latter by edge effects.

HIGHER-ORDER NEAREST NEIGHBOR ANALYSIS

The occurrence of more than a single process may occur, for example, when pairs tend to couple together while another process may or may not be present.

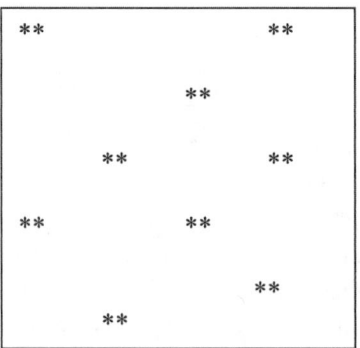

FIGURE 7.2   Illustration of pairwise clustering in a dispersed population.

The resulting interpretation may miss the pairwise, or higher-order, clustering. This could be avoided by examining, in addition to the nearest neighbor, distances between second, or higher-order, closest points. The order selected depends on the particular problem being examined. Regardless of the order, the Z statistic is calculated similarly. In addition, constants for the mean distance and standard deviation coefficients in eqq. (3) and (5) will be added to reflect the order tested. The constants for k^{th}-order neighbor calculations were derived by Dacey and Tung (1962) and appear in Figure 7.1.

The calculation of the expected distance to the kth-nearest neighbor was derived by Thompson (1965) as

$$\overline{D}_{ran} = \frac{1}{\sqrt{N/A}} \frac{k(2k)!}{(2^k k!)^2},$$ (7)

where k = the order of the nearest neighbor.

For example, if $k = 2$,

$$\overline{D}_{ran} = \frac{1}{\sqrt{N/A}} \frac{2(2 \times 2)!}{(2^2 2!)^2} = \frac{1}{\sqrt{N/A}} \frac{2 \times 4 \times 3 \times 2 \times 1}{8^2} = \frac{0.75}{\sqrt{N/A}}.$$ (d)

Table 7.1 illustrates examples of charts for alternative point distributions.

CUZICK-EDWARDS' TEST

One problem associated with the nearest neighbor test is that it does not adjust for a population at risk that is not randomly distributed. The result is that the test result of a subset, for example, cases or outbreak premises, of this population will be biased toward the underlying distribution of the population at risk. For example, animal populations, whether companion, livestock, or wildlife, tend to be clustered either around or outside of human populations. To adjust for the nonhomogeneous (inhomogeneous) or non-Poisson distribution of the population at risk, a number of alternatives to the nearest neighbor method

TABLE 7.1   Constants Used in the Calculation of Mean and Standard Deviation of Distance Measures

Order of neighbor	Mean distance coefficient*	Standard deviation coefficient
1	0.5000	0.26136
2	0.7500	0.27221
3	0.9375	0.27568
4	1.0975	0.27749
5	1.2305	0.27839
6	1.3535	0.27893

*Calculated from the equation $\frac{k(2k)!}{(2^k k!)^2}$.

have been used. Bithell (1990) estimated a relative risk function for childhood leukemia in Cumbria, United Kingdom, comparing first- and second-nearest neighbor distances for cases and randomly selected controls. A similar approach was taken by Gatrell and Bailey (1996), who estimated K functions for randomly selected cases and controls of childhood leukemia in Lancashire, United Kingdom. They examined the difference plots of these two functions against distance. Significant clustering is identified when peaks exceed an analytic or simulated confidence interval (CI). Glaser (1990) used two alternative techniques, one of which adjusts for population density algebraically (Whittemore et al. 1987), whereas the second produces a transformed map in which the population is uniformly distributed (Selvin 1996) to examine clustering of Hogkin's disease in the San Francisco Bay area. The most commonly used approach to control for the distribution of the population at risk was developed by Cuzick and Edwards (1990). They use a variation of the kth-nearest neighbor approach whereby cases are examined with respect to their number of nearest neighbors that are also cases. The expected number of nearest neighbors that are cases is based on the number and proportion of cases in the case-control selection. In contrast to the traditional nearest neighbor test, the Cuzick-Edwards' test considers the relative and not actual distance between points. Kulldorf and Nagarwalla (1995) adapted the scan test for application to nonhomogeneously distributed spatial data. All of these techniques control for the bias toward clustering that one typically finds with the basic nearest neighbor test.

The Cuzick-Edwards' test is a one-tailed, nonparametric test based on the number of cases among the k nearest neighbors of each case nearer than the k nearest controls. The locations of each of the z_i points are given by the x_i,y_i coordinates. For each case, the number of cases (n_0) that are k^{th}-nearest neighbors is determined (by Euclidean distance) and compared with the expected number. For example, in Figure 7.3, there are seven cases and eight controls. The number of cases having another case as its first-nearest neighbors in this illustration is four (points 1, 5, 6 and 7), as illustrated by the arrows. Note that points 6 and 7 are reflexive points—they are each other's first-nearest neighbor—and therefore count twice in the sum of the total number of cases that have cases as first-nearest neighbors. The expected number of cases being first-nearest neighbors for the seven cases is calculated as

$$E(T_k) = pkn, \tag{8}$$

where

$$p = \frac{n_0}{n} \frac{n_0 - 1}{n - 1}. \tag{9}$$

Thus, in the example presented in Figure 7.3, $p = (7/15)(6/14) = 0.2$. It follows that the expected number of first-nearest neighbors being cases for the

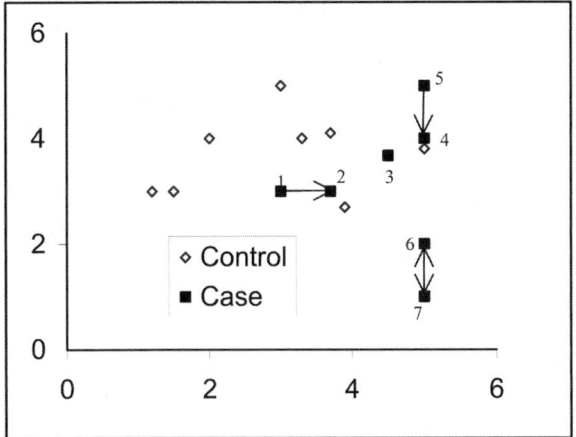

FIGURE 7.3   Hypothetical point distribution to illustrate the Cuzick-Edwards' test.

cases is $E(T_k) = 0.2 \times 1 \times 14 = 3$. Similarly, the expected number of cases being either the first or second-nearest neighbors for the cases is six, and so on for higher-order nearest neighbors.

The variance is calculated as

$$V(T_k) = (kn + N_s)p_1(1 - p_1) + [3(k^2 - k)n + N_t - 2N_s](p_2 - p_1^2)$$
$$- [k^2(n^2 - 3n) + N_s - N_t](p_1^2 - p_3), \tag{10}$$

where

$$Ns = \sum_i \sum_j a_{ij}a_{ji}, \tag{11}$$

which is equal to two times the number of reciprocal nearest neighbor pairs, and

$$Nt = \sum_{i \neq l} \sum \sum a_{ij}a_{lj}, \tag{12}$$

which is the number of points that are the nearest neighbor to two other points. Further, for $k > 1$,

$$p_k = p_{k-1}\frac{n_0 - k}{n - k}. \tag{13}$$

Thus,

$$p_2 = p\frac{n_0 - 2}{n - 2}, \tag{e}$$

and

TABLE 7.2   Estimates used for N_s/n and N_t/n

K	N_s/n	N_t/n
1	0.6215	0.6332
2	1.4211	3.1737
3	2.2731	7.6969
4	3.1503	14.2159
5	4.0431	22.7355
6	4.9468	33.2505

Note. From Cuzick and Edwards 1990.

$$p_3 = p_2 \frac{n_0 - 3}{n - 3} \tag{f}$$

Estimates for N_s and N_t have been made by Cuzick and Edwards and are presented in Table 7.2.

In this example, the variance for the $E(T_k)$ is 2.26. The significance test uses the Z statistic:

$$Z = \frac{E(Tk) - Tk}{\sqrt{\mathrm{var}(Tk)}}. \tag{14}$$

Therefore, in this example, the cases are more clustered (four nearest neighbors observed) than expected (three cases); that is, $T_k > E(T_k)$. The associated Z statistic shows that this pattern is not significantly ($P = .25$) different from random.

$$Z = \frac{4 - 3}{\sqrt{2.26}} = 0.67. \tag{g}$$

CASE STUDIES

CANINE LEPTOSPIROSIS IN INDIANA

Leptospirosis is a serious disease in dogs, with reported case-fatality rates ranging from 10% to 20%. It is characterized by acute renal and hepatic failure and coagulation abnormalities. Leptospirosis is caused by many different *Leptospira* serovars. Reservoirs of *Leptospira* serovars may vary in different parts of the world. Following introduction of a bivalent vaccine against serovars canicola and icterohaemmorrhagiae in the early 1970s, the incidence of leptospirosis in dogs in the United States decreased. However, beginning in the early 1980s, the prevalence of canine leptosirosis has been increasing (Ward et al. 2002). Many of these cases are apparently caused by serovar grippotyphosa, which has wildlife species as maintenance hosts. More opportunity for contact between dogs and wildlife, such as skunks, raccoons, and opossums, caused by expansion of urban areas into wildlife habitats may be a reason for the epidemic of leptospirosis in the United States (Bolin 1996). On a national basis, clustering of canine leptospirosis in the United States has been described (Ward 2002a), as has its relationship with rainfall (Ward 2002b).

The Veterinary Medical Data Base (VMDB) was used to identify records of dogs examined at the Purdue University veterinary teaching hospital between January 1, 1997, and December 31, 2002, that were diagnosed as clinical cases of leptospirosis (VMDB diagnosis code 010017200). A total of 39 cases of leptospirosis were identified (249 cases per 100,000 dogs examined; 95% CI, 179 to 343). The highest serovar-specific rates were estimated for serovars grippotyphosa (134 per 100,000 dogs examined; 95% CI, 85 to 209) and bratislava (51 per 100,000 dogs examined; 95% CI, 24 to 105). During the same period, 138 dogs (controls) were identified that had been admitted to the Purdue University veterinary teaching hospital and had been tested negative (microscopic agglutination test $<$ 1:100) for leptospirosis.

The location of cases and controls was identified by using the Zip code of the address of the owner of each dog and the longitude and latitiude of the centroid of Zip codes (Figures 7.4 and 7.5). The results of the nearest neighbor test

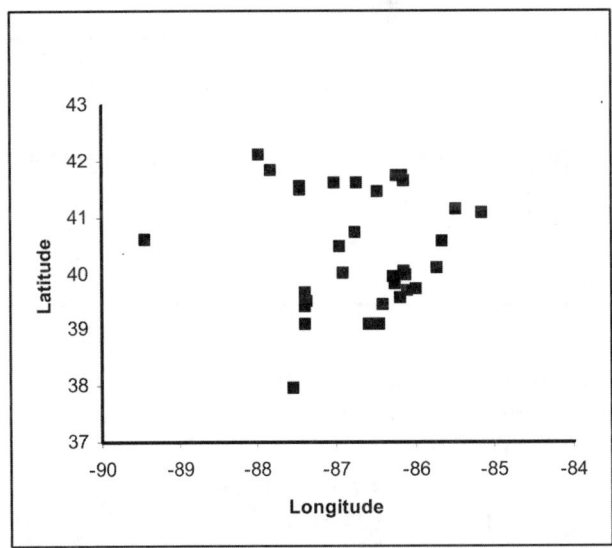

FIGURE 7.4   Spatial distribution of canine leptospirosis cases reported diagnosed at Purdue University veterinary teaching hospital, 1997 to 2002.

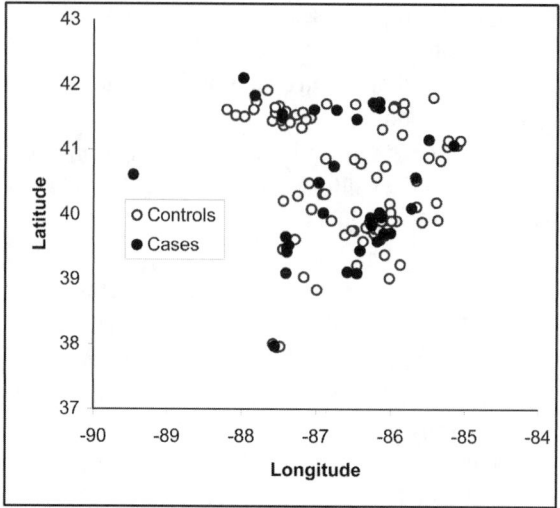

FIGURE 7.5   Spatial distribution of canine leptospirosis cases and controls diagnosed at Purdue University veterinary teaching hospital, 1997 to 2002.

TABLE 7.3   Results of the Nearest-Neighbor Test of the Distribution of Canine Leptospirosis Cases Diagnosed at Purdue University Veterinary Teaching Hospital, 1997 to 2002

K^{th} neighbor	1	2	3	4	5	6
$\overline{D}_{obs}$	0.213	0.304	0.360	0.455	0.547	0.610
D_{ran}	0.338	0.507	0.634	0.742	0.832	0.915
Index	0. 632	0.600	0.567	0.614	0.658	0.667
Standard error	0.0060	0.0063	0.0064	0.0064	0.0064	0.0064
Z statistic	−13.19	−20.55	−23.32	−27.57	−29.87	−33.70
Area	12.43					
Density	12.31					

of the distribution of canine leptospirosis cases is shown in Table 7.3. At all nearest neighbor orders examined (1 through 6), there was significant ($P < .01$) evidence of clustering of cases ($R = 0.57$ to 0.67). The results of the Cuzick and Edwards' test are shown in Table 7.4. In contrast to the nearest neighbor test analysis of cases of leptopsirosis, no significant ($P > .24$) evidence of clustering was detected using the Cuzick and Edwards' test.

In this example, a referral hospital was used to identify cases of leptspirosis. Controls were dogs presented at the same hospital and that tested negative for

TABLE 7.4   Results of the Cuzick-Edwards' test of the Distribution of Canine Leptospirosis Cases Diagnosed at Purdue University Veterinary Teaching Hospital, 1997 to 2002

K^{th} neighbor	1	2	3	4	5	6
T_k	6	13	19	29	34	45
$E(T_k)$	7.8	15.6	23.4	31.2	39	46.8
$V(T_k)$	9.54	19.47	29.22	38.80	48.65	57.95
Z statistic	0.58	0.59	0.81	0.35	0.72	0.24

leptospirosis. These dogs were presented with signs suggestive of leptospirosis and were tested to rule out the disease. As for all hospital-based studies, a geographically defined source population exists from which patients are presented at the hospital. Such populations tend to be closer to the hospital and get smaller as the distance from the hospital increases. In addition, for human and companion animal populations, the presence of major metropolitan areas (e.g., Indianapolis and East Chicago in Indiana) skews this source population distribution. The skewness in the source population is likely to be responsible for the spatial clustering detected in the nearest neighbor analysis, even in the absence of variables that might result in the clustering of leptospirosis. The inhomogeneity in the population is accounted for in the Cuzick and Edwards' test analysis by sampling controls from the same population using the dogs presented at the same veterinary hospital. Thus, cases and controls represent the spatial distribution of the source population. Given the location of the control dogs presented to the hospital, there is no evidence that cases presented to the same hospital are spatially clustered.

FOWL CHOLERA IN CALIFORNIA

Fowl cholera (FC) is one of the most economically important diseases facing the turkey industry in the United States, including in California. A cooperative effort between the California Turkey Federation and epidemiologists and microbiologists was undertaken to better understand the epidemiology of this disease and, ultimately, its effect on the turkey industry. To do this, we combined multivariable statistical techniques with modern epidemiologic fingerprinting and cluster detection techniques (Carpenter et al. 1991, 1996). In this chapter, we will report the techniques used and the findings obtained in the cluster detection portion of the study.

From 1985 through 1986, a total of 49 outbreaks of fowl cholera were reported in California turkey flocks (Figure 7.6). One of the hypotheses examined to better understand the mode of flock-to-flock transmission was that an

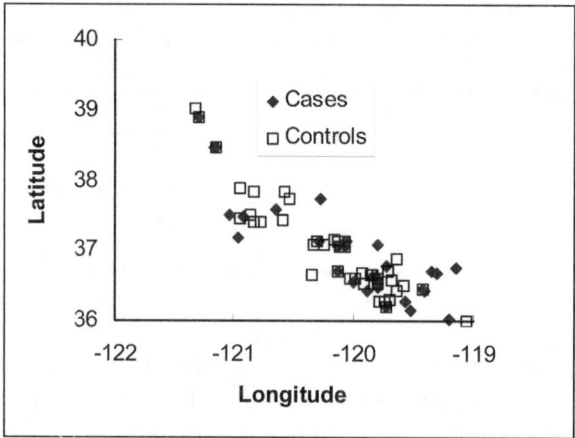

FIGURE 7.6   Spatial distribution of turkey premises infected with fowl cholera in California, 1985 to 1986.

insufficient biosecurity was involved. If inadequate biosecurity were responsible for transmitting the infection between flocks, we expected that FC outbreak flocks would be spatially clustered. To test this assumption, we applied the nearest neighbor test to the outbreak data. Results of the nearest neighbor test are presented in Table 7.5, for the sixth-nearest neighbors. There is a consistent pattern in that the observed nearest neighbor distance is approximately 0.4 (see index values; i.e., $\overline{D}_{\text{obs}}/\overline{D}_{\text{ran}}$)—what would be expected if these points were randomly distributed throughout the study region. However, as is often the case with livestock, premises tend to be clustered regardless of dis-

TABLE 7.5   **Results of the Nearest-Neighbor Test of the Distribution of Fowl Cholera-Infected Turkey Premises, 1985 to 1986.**

K^{th} neighbor	1	2	3	4	5	6
$\overline{D}_{\text{obs}}$	0.608	0.872	1.040	1.299	1.400	1.595
$\overline{D}_{\text{ran}}$	1.410	2.115	2.643	3.094	3.469	3.816
Index	0.432	0.412	0.393	0.420	0.403	0.418
Standard error	0.0132	0.0138	0.0140	0.0141	0.0141	0.0141
Z statistic	−7.61	−11.33	−14.44	−16.07	−18.42	−19.77
Area	6.16					
Density	7.95					

ease status. If this were true, ignoring the inherent clustering in the underlying population will bias findings toward clustering of FC. It is, therefore, necessary to examine and adjust for the distribution of the population at risk before analyzing a sample, for example, cases, of that population.

As discussed above, one test that adjusts for the nonrandom, or inhomogeneous, distribution of a population is the Cuzick-Edwards' test. We examined the distribution of the 49 cases (FC-infected or outbreak premises) when considered as part of the total turkey population in the study area. To do this, we obtained the geographic location of a random sample of 43 control (nonoutbreak) premises. Our findings were consistent with those observed when we examined the case data alone using the nearest neighbor test (Table 7.6). That is, after adjusting for the nonrandom distribution of the population of turkey premises, cases (outbreak premises) remained significantly clustered ($.01 < P < .05$). This information supported our hypothesis that meat bird turkey premises were at increased risk of becoming infected with fowl cholera if a similar neighboring premise were also infected. It also supported a hypothesis that meat bird flocks lacked adequate biosecurity measures to safeguard against frequent contact with the various work crews that traveled among these premises. As a result of our findings, the turkey industry increased biosecurity measures and the incidence of fowl cholera similarly decreased.

PRECAUTIONS

It should be noted that spatial-cluster tests are sensitive and potentially biased because of nonhomogeneous distributions of the population at-risk dynamics. Ignoring this may result in biased findings. We have demonstrated how this bias may be overcome if the population is nonhomogeneously distributed. Another bias may be introduced if the distribution of the population at risk is not stable. Similarly, recognition and reporting bias should be ruled out as possible explanations for spatial clustering.

TABLE 7.6 Results of the Cuzick-Edwards' Test of the Distribution of Fowl Cholera-Infected Turkey Premises, 1985 to 1986.

K^{th} neighbor	1	2	3	4	5	6
$E(T_k)$	25.8	51.7	77.5	103.4	129.2	155.1
T_k	32	61	93	118	147	176
$V(T_k)$	14.16	26.88	43.14	62.09	82.56	106.91
Z statistic	1.64	1.80	2.35	1.85	1.96	2.02

CONCLUSIONS

In conclusion, detection of a spatial cluster of events such as disease or illness is one of many steps that may assist us in identifying causes of disease and suggesting effective methods of control. In addition, other statistical tests, including traditional statistical tests such as regression, may be used independently or in combination with temporal, spatial, and temporal-spatial tests to improve the understanding of complex systems associated with these events. A better understanding and more frequent application of these tools should help epidemiologists and others involved with disease control to do their jobs more effectively.

BIBLIOGRAPHY

Alexander F.E., Boyle P. (Eds.). 1996. *Methods for Investigating Localized Clustering of Disease*, IARC Scientific Publications no. 135, Lyon, France: International Agency for Research on Cancer, World Health Organization.

Armitage P., Berry G. 1994. Statistical methods in medical research, 3rd ed. Blackwell Scientific, Oxford, pp 530–533.

Bithell J.F. 1990. An application of density estimation to geographical epidemiology. Stat Med 9:691–701.

Bolin C.A. 1996. Diagnosis of leptospirosis: A reemerging disease of companion animals. Semin Vet Med Surg Small Anim 11:166–171.

Carpenter T.E. 2001. Methods to investigate spatial and temporal clustering in veterinary epidemiology. Prev Vet Med 48:303–320.

Carpenter T.E., Hird D.W., Snipes K.P. 1996. A time-space investigation of the epidemiology of fowl cholera. Prev Vet Med 28:159–163.

Carpenter T.E., Snipes K.P., Kasten R.W., Hird D.W., Hirsh D.C. 1991. Molecular epidemiology of *Pasteurella multocida*. Am J Vet Res 52:1345–1349.

Clark P.J., Evans F.C. 1954. Distance to nearest neighbor as a measure of spatial relationships in populations. Ecology 35:445–453.

Cliff A.D., Ord J.K. 1981. Spatial processes, models and applications. Pion, London.

Cuzick J., Edwards R. 1990. Spatial clustering for inhomogeneous populations. J R Stat Soc B 52:73–104.

Dacey M.F., Tung T.H. 1962. The identification of randomness in point patterns. J Reg Sci 4:83–96.

Davis J.C. 1986. Statistics and data analysis in geology, 2nd ed. Wiley, New York.

Earickson R.J., Harlin J.M. 1994. Geographic measurement and quantitative analysis, Macmillan College, New York.

Ebdon D. 1985. Statistics in geography: A practical approach, 2nd ed. Basil Blackwell, New York.

Elliot P., Cuzick J., English D., Stern D. (Eds.). 1992. Geographical and environmental epidemiology: Methods for small-area studies. Oxford University Press, Oxford.

Gatrell A.C., Bailey T.C. 1996. Interactive spatial data analysis in medical geography. Soc Sci Med 42:843–855.

Glaser S.L. 1990. Spatial clustering of Hodgkin's disease in San Francisco Bay area. Am J Epidemiol 132:S167-S177.

Haining R. 1990. Spatial data analysis in the social and environmental sciences, Cambridge University Press, Cambridge.

Jacquez G.M., Grimson R., Waller L.A., Wartenberg D. 1996a. On disease clustering part II: Introduction to techniques. Inf Control Hosp Epidemiol 17:385–397.

Jacquez G.M., Waller L.A., Grimson R., Wartenberg D. 1996b. On disease clustering part I: State of the art. Inf Control Hosp Epidemiol 17:319–327.

Krebs C.J. 1999. Ecological methodology, 2nd ed. Benjamin/Cummings, Menlo Park, NJ.

Kulldorf M., Nagarwalla N. 1995. Spatial disease clusters: Detection and inference. Stat Med 14:799–810.

Lawson A.B. 2001. Statistical methods in spatial epidemiology, Wiley, New York.

McGlashan N.D. (Ed.). 1972. Medical geography: Techniques and field studies. Methuen, London.

Moore D.A., Carpenter T.E. 1999. Spatial analytic methods and geographic information systems: Use in health research and epidemiology. Epidemiol Rev 21:143–161.

Ripley B.D. 1988. Statistical inference for spatial processes. Cambridge University Press, Cambridge.

Selvin S. 1996. Statistical analysis of epidemiological data, 2nd ed. Oxford University Press, New York.

Thomas R.W. (Ed.). 1990. Spatial epidemiology. London Papers in Regional Science 21. Pion, London.

Thompson H.R. 1965. Distribution of distance to Nth neighbour in a population of randomly distributed individuals. Ecology 37:391–394.

Upton G.J.G., Fingleton B. 1985. Spatial data analysis by example: Point pattern and quantitative data. Wiley, New York.

Ward M.P. 2002a. Clustering of leptospirosis among dogs in the United States and Canada. Prev Vet Med 56:215–226

Ward M.P. 2002b. Seasonality of canine leptospirosis in the United States and Canada and its association with rainfall. Prev Vet Med 56:203–213.

Ward M.P., Carpenter T.E. 2000a. Analysis of time-space clustering in veterinary epidemiology. Prev Vet Med 43:225–237.

Ward M.P., Carpenter T.E. 2000b. Techniques for analysing the clustering of disease in space and in time in veterinary epidemiology. Prev Vet Med 45:257–284.

Ward M.P., Glickman L.T., Guptill L.F. 2002. Prevalence of and risk factors for leptospirosis among dogs in the United States and Canada: 677 cases. JAVMA 220:53–58.

Whittemore A.S., Friend N., Brown B.W., Holly E.A. 1987. A test to detect clusters of disease. Biometrika 74:631–635.

Use of Sentinel Herds in Monitoring and Surveillance Systems

B.J. McCluskey

INTRODUCTION

Sentinel surveillance is used to monitor or identify outbreaks and epidemics caused by infectious agents, to investigate changes in the prevalence or incidence of endemic diseases or infectious agents, to evaluate the effectiveness of newly instituted disease control programs, and to confirm a hypothesis about the ecology or epidemiology of an infectious agent. This concept is one in which the health status of populations is periodically assessed. Sentinel surveillance has been applied liberally in development of public health surveillance systems (Parrish and McDonnell 1994; Thacker et al., 1983). Applications of sentinel surveillance for animal health, although infrequent, have generally been successful.

United States Department of Agriculture
Centers for Epidemiology and Animal Health
2150 Centre Avenue
Building B
Fort Collins, CO, 80526

Public health applications of sentinel surveillance have been used to monitor or identify epidemics of infectious diseases or to monitor the activity of conditions, such as asthma, that change because of environmental conditions. These systems cannot measure the magnitude of disease incidence or prevalence, as they are not population based. Accurate incidence and prevalence estimates require knowledge of the population at risk for which the estimate is made. The French Communicable Disease Network (Sentiweb) has linked physicians in general practice throughout France by terminals supplied by the telephone company or through an Internet website (Valleron and Garnerin 1992). The United States Influenza Sentinel Physicians Surveillance Network enlists approximately 260 physicians around the country who provide weekly reports on the total number of patients seen and the number of those patients with influenza-like illness by age group. Other sentinel systems employing physicians, hospitals, and laboratories reporting on a variety of diseases or identification of disease agents exist in the United States and in other countries.

The list of sentinel surveillance systems in animal health is much shorter. The most well-known and developed animal health sentinel surveillance system is the National Arbovirus Monitoring Program (NAMP) in Australia (Animal Health Australia 2001). NAMP is a program managed by Animal Health Australia, a public company formed by the commonwealth, state, and territory ministers of agriculture and the presidents of the national councils of Australia's livestock industries. The NAMP is funded by the industry and government agencies, and its goal is to monitor the distribution of certain arthropod-borne livestock viruses and their vectors. The viruses of interest include Akabane, bluetongue virus (BTV), and bovine ephemeral fever viruses. Data for this system are collected in sentinel cattle herds throughout Australia. Ten or more immunologically naïve young cattle on each sentinel location are blood tested at prescribed intervals to detect seroconversion to the viruses. Additional details of this system will be presented in later sections of this chapter.

In Canada, sentinel herds are also employed for BTV surveillance. Five sites were established in the Okanogan Valley of British Colombia in 1988. These sites were chosen because they had been identified to historically experience incursions of BTV (Kellar 1999). A consortium of government agencies, producer groups, and a university in Canada also established the sentinel herd mastitis project. This project used 27 sentinel veterinary practices, 40 veterinarians, and 60 dairy herds to investigate the incidence of mastitis and monitor changes in incidence and management practices on dairies in Ontario (Kellar 1999).

A sentinel system that bridges public health and animal health surveillance is exemplified by surveillance for West Nile virus. Live-bird surveillance, usually sentinel chicken flocks, has historically been used to both detect and monitor arboviral diseases, including St. Louis encephalitis, eastern equine encephalitis, and western equine encephalitis. Recently this approach has been applied to surveillance for West Nile virus, which affects both humans and livestock. The U.S. Centers for Disease Control and Prevention states that captive bird sentinel surveillance must use a species that is universally susceptible to infection to the agent of interest, that must survive the infection and develop easily detectable antibodies, that poses no risk of infection to handlers, and that never develops sufficient viremia that potential arthropod vectors might become infected.

No doubt there are additional examples of sentinel surveillance systems or projects initiated by animal health officials or academic institutions in many countries. The purpose of this chapter is to provide guidance in the establishment of sentinel surveillance systems. The rationale and limitations of these systems are discussed in addition to specific procedures necessary for their implementation.

RATIONALE FOR SENTINEL SURVEILLANCE

The need for and uses of animal health surveillance are addressed in Chapters 1 and 2 of this book. Improvements in animal health and livestock production and direction in appropriately allocating normally limited resources are all-encompassing goals of surveillance. The international expectations of scientifically based disease risk management strategies require accurate and timely surveillance data.

Many countries have government-sponsored systems for the routine collection of animal health information. Systems may include requirements for routine testing of all herds for a particular disease agent or testing of animals at slaughter. Determining how many animals are in how many herds in a specific geographic area to provide some statistically estimable level of confidence that the disease does not exist or that it exists at some predetermined level has been the difficult task of many veterinary epidemiologists and biostatisticians in the last few years. In most cases, the number of animals and herds required are large, resulting in substantial investment of animal health resources. Surveillance systems are also implemented to monitor changes in occurrence of disease by time, place, species, and other host characteristics. Sentinel surveillance systems have been of greatest value for this application because of their ability to do targeted sampling and reduce costs.

Sentinel surveillance promotes targeting of herds or areas with higher probabilities of disease. Prior knowledge of disease distribution allows surveillance activities to focus on the margins of disease-free and endemic areas or the borders between high- and low-prevalence areas. Absence of prior knowledge of disease distribution would necessitate a more random distribution of sentinel herds.

The cost effectiveness of sentinel surveillance systems makes them an attractive alternative to slaughter surveillance and cross-sectional surveys in situations in which sentinel surveillance systems are an appropriate option. Slaughter surveillance systems sample animals at the time of slaughter, with subsequent testing of samples for antibodies to disease agents of interest, for the disease agents themselves, or for residues. The United States Department of Agriculture (USDA)'s Animal and Plant Health Inspection Service, Veterinary Services, estimates per animal collection and testing costs for bovine brucellosis slaughter surveillance to range from US$.60 to US$1.50 (M. Gilsdorf, personal communication). An estimated 12 million samples from test-eligible animals are required to achieve program goals and to reach predetermined statistically valid estimates of disease prevalence resulting in total slaughter surveillance costs of US$7.2–18 million. Slaughter surveillance for bovine tuberculosis has estimated per animal sampling and testing costs between US$31 and US$34 and total annual testing costs ranging from US$124,000 to US$127,000.

Population-based surveys with random sampling are similarly expensive and often difficult to conduct if adequate list frames of livestock and poultry operations are not available. Surveys generally provide one time sampling (point estimates), thus requiring that they be repeated to assess changes in disease prevalence.

ESTABLISHING SENTINEL SURVEILLANCE

HERD OR SITE SELECTION

Goals of the sentinel system under consideration will certainly influence how herds or sites are selected. In the case of the National Arbovirus Monitoring Program in Australia, the primary goal is to facilitate plotting of the distribution of arboviral infections in cattle (Animal Health Australia 2001). At first, herds were selected to provide a random distribution throughout the country. True random selection of herds requires a deliberate process in which each herd has an equal probability of being selected (Thrusfield 1995). This type of sampling uses a "list" of all herds in the population that meet the criteria of the study and a random number generator to assist in selection. In the NAMP, site selection now depends largely on the availability and interest of the regulatory field veterinarian in the area and the willingness of the operation's owner (Table 8.1). Sentinel surveillance requires repeated visits to the sentinel sites

Table 8.1   National Arbovirus Monitoring Program: Numbers of Sites and Collections, 1999 through 2000

| | Serology and/or virology | | | | | |
| | Bluetongue | | Akabane | | Ephemeral fever | |
State/territory	Sites	Collections	Sites	Collections	Sites	Collections
New South Wales	31	123	31	123	31	123
Northern Territory	14	97	13	97	13	97
Queensland	23	76	23	71	23	71
South Australia	4	8	4	8	1	2
Tasmania	3	6	3	6	3	6
Victoria	5	10	5	10	5	10
Western Australia	10	30	10	31	10	30

Note. Used with permission from Dr. M.J. Nunn, Manager (Animal Health Science), Office of the Chief Veterinary Officer, Agriculture, Fisheries and Forestry, Australia.

and, consequently, a commitment from the operations owner to allow such visits or to allow regulatory authority to make such visits. Incentives to operation owners, including cash compensation or free or reduced cost of diagnostic testing, may help in retention of sentinel surveillance sites.

As mentioned previously, targeting of surveillance is an advantage of sentinel surveillance and may affect site selection. The longevity of the NAMP in Australia has provided data indicating viral distribution so that program coordinators can locate sites where previous viral activity has occurred along the margins of previous viral activity to detect incursions of virus into new areas and in "free" areas to ensure they remain "free" areas.

Determining how many herds or operations to include in a sentinel system again depends on the goals of the system and, in many situations, on available resources. Using sentinel herds to determine freedom from a particular infectious agent in a specific geographical area is a valid approach. Determining sample size estimates for various types of surveillance is discussed in Chapter 4.

ANIMAL SELECTION

How many and which animals to include as sentinels is an important consideration when developing sentinel surveillance systems. The sentinel animals selected must be susceptible to the infectious agent and generate a measurable clinical or immunological response. A cohort of young, immunologically naïve animals often make the ideal sentinels, although adult animals may also be used. If young animals are to be marketed after initial sampling, they would not be the best choice for sentinels. Although cohorts are followed through time, sentinel surveillance is different from a cohort study. A cohort study is designed to find risk factors associated with the occurrence of disease by following two separate groups of individuals: one group with exposures to suspected risk factors, and one group without these exposures. Cohorts used in sentinel systems are used as disease detectors, and although risk factors of disease can be assessed, disease monitoring is the primary purpose of the cohorts. The sentinel animals chosen should be available for examination or sampling at each visit to monitor responses to the agent. This requirement often results in the owner of the operation choosing sentinel animals by convenience; that is, those that can be made available at each visit or those that can be easily handled. Because the herd is the unit of observation, not the individual animal, random selection of sentinel animals is not imperative as long as those chosen are susceptible and likely to be exposed to the agent if it is present on the site.

Sample size estimates for sentinels on each site are based on standard formulas for detection of disease at predetermined prevalences and confidence levels. FreeCalc is a free software package that assists in the planning and analysis of surveys to detect disease or prove freedom from disease (Cameron and Baldock 1998). FreeCalc calculates sample size requirements based on diagnostic test sensitivity and specificity, taking population size into account, and can be used to determine the number of sentinel animals required on each site. Sample size estimates must be increased by a factor that accounts for the likelihood of dropouts. Sentinel animals may be sold, die, or no longer be available for other reasons and thus be lost to follow-up sampling.

FREQUENCY OF SAMPLING

The frequency of sentinel site visits and subsequent sampling of sentinel animals is based on the goals of the surveillance and on the biology of the infectious agent of interest. Table 8.2 suggests sampling frequency of sentinel sites by the various frequencies of disease occurrence and by the effects the occurrence may have on animal populations. These effects may be direct (e.g., loss of production or death) or indirect (i.e., restrictions on trade of live animals or animal products).

As mentioned previously, sampling frequency is also determined by the biology of the infectious agent. For example, transmission of BTV occurs almost exclusively by species of Culicoides. In the United States, subspecies of *Culicoides varipennis* are the primary vectors. These vectors hatch, feed, and breed from March through October, with peak activity in June through September.

TABLE 8.2   Suggested Frequency of Sampling for Sentinel Herd Surveillance Applications

Disease occurrence	Disease effect	Example	Sampling frequency
Very rare	Severe	Foot and Mouth Disease in a nearby country	Weekly
Rare	Severe	Bovine brucellosis in free countries	Annually
Sporadic	Severe	Neosporosis outbreaks	Quarterly
Sporadic	Moderate	Vesicular stomatitis in the southwest United States	Semiannually
Endemic	Severe	Bluetongue in endemic countries	Semiannually
Endemic	Moderate	Vesicular stomatitis in Central America	Annually

Monitoring transmission of BTV through sentinel surveillance should most appropriately occur during the months of vector activity.

Sentinel sites used for research purposes could be sampled more or less often than suggested in Table 8.2, depending on the infectious agent under investigation and on the resources available for the study.

TESTING

Assessment of a sentinel animal's response to the infectious agent of interest is accomplished through clinical examination, serological testing, or identification of the infectious agent itself. Using clinical examinations as the sole determinant of a positive sentinel animal is tenuous. Different infectious agents may express very similar clinical manifestations (e.g., foot and mouth disease and vesicular stomatitis), requiring more specific discernment than a clinical examination can provide.

Various serological procedures to detect antibodies to infectious agents are available including numerous ELISA techniques, serum neutralization assays, complement fixation tests, agglutination tests, and many others. Availability is dependent on the infectious agent of interest. Immunologically naïve animals would be expected to respond to the disease agent of interest in a measurable way. The primary immune response would be measurable by most, if not all, of the available serologic tests for that agent. However, animals already positive by one or more of the serological tests need not be excluded as sentinel animals. Many assays can detect immunoglobulins of the IgM class. These antibodies are usually the earliest antibodies to be detectable after an antigenic stimulus but tend to decline rapidly and then disappear. Reinfection with the identical agent may stimulate a new, measurable IgM response. Serological tests that allow quantification of the amount of antibody can also be useful in animals previously exposed to the agent of interest. It is generally accepted that a fourfold rise in antibody titer indicates recent exposure to an infectious agent. For some agents this may indicate a recrudescence of a latent pathogen, and for others, re-exposure to the pathogen by the environment or other infected animals.

Isolation of the agent of interest or detection of genetic material from the agent (e.g., polymerase chain reaction techniques) from sentinel animals or from the environment of the sentinel site provides the best indication of the presence of the agent, although these techniques are often the most expensive and difficult to conduct.

EXAMPLES

To highlight the steps necessary in developing sentinel surveillance systems, two examples of sentinel herd projects will follow. In both examples the infectious agents of interest are vesicular stomatitis viruses.

Vesicular stomatitis viruses affect cattle, pigs and horses (McCluskey et al. 1999), and there are two serotypes of concern, vesicular stomatitis virus–New Jersey (VSV-NJ) and vesicular stomatitis virus–Indiana (VSV-IN). Clinical signs of disease may include vesicles and erosions of the oral and nasal mucosa, coronitis, vesicles or erosions of the udder and teats, and crusting lesions of the muzzle, ventral abdomen, and external genitalia. Vesicular stomatitis (VS) is endemic in South America, Central America, and parts of Mexico and on Ossabaw Island, a small barrier island off the coast of the state of Georgia in the United States. The disease has been considered epidemic in the southwestern United States with sporadic outbreaks of VS occurring in this region. Outbreaks appear to be associated with arthropod transmission of the virus. Researchers with the Animal Population Health Institute at Colorado State University and the USDA's Centers for Epidemiology and Animal Health hypothesized that vesicular stomatitis viruses were present in the southwestern United States in nonoutbreak years and determined that the best way to test this hypothesis was through sentinel herd testing of operations in the southwestern United States as well as using operations in endemic areas of Central America as a comparison group.

SENTINEL HERDS IN EL SALVADOR

A total of 14 sentinel farms were selected from four different regions of El Salvador. These farms were selected on the basis of samples of farms that were confirmed to have housed VS-positive cattle in one or more outbreaks during the years 1997 through 2000 or that were adjacent to farms with positive cases during the outbreaks. These farms must have housed at least 20 dairy cows. Vesicular cases must have been confirmed as positive by the presence of clinical signs of VS and positive virus isolation or positive serologic test results. The confirmed positive cases did not necessarily still reside on the farms at the initiation of the sentinel study.

The distribution of the farms by regions was as follows (Figure 8.1): the Department of Sonsonate, four farms; the Department of Chalatenango, six farms (two dropped out from the study); the Department of San Miguel, two farms; the Department of La Union, two farms.

The selection of the sentinel cohorts was based on the population of cows on each farm. All heifers from 6 to 12 months of age were sampled from those farms with 30 or fewer heifers. On dairies with more than 30 cows, 15% of their additional heifers (above 30) were sampled.

The farms' owners were required to commit to a minimum of two years of participation in the study and to monthly collection of biological samples from a cohort of cattle. Those farms having more than one susceptible animal species (equine, swine, or bovine) or neighboring a farm with other species were preferentially selected to participate in the study.

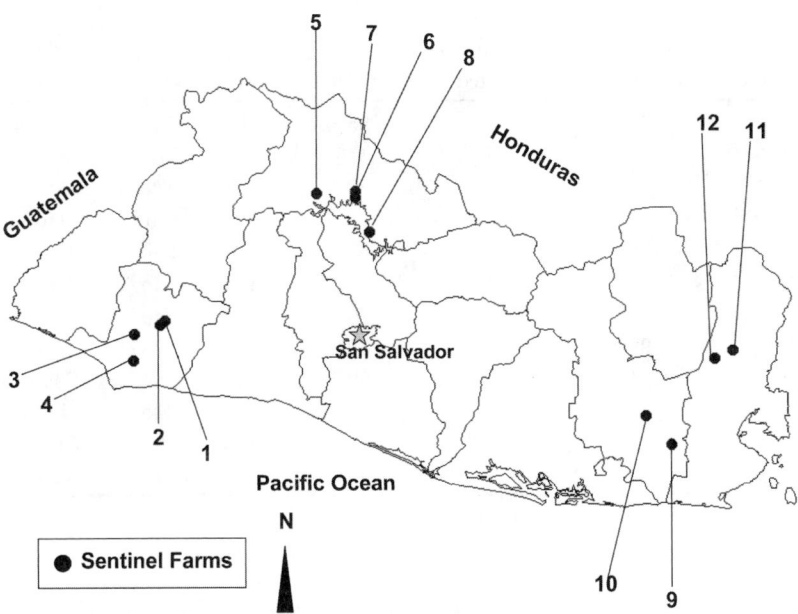

FIGURE 8.1   Distribution of the farms by regions in El Salvador.

Biological samples were collected monthly from heifers enrolled in the study. A serum sample and oral swab were collected from each heifer. At the same time, an examination of the oral cavity, nasal mucosa, coronary bands, mammary glands, and genitalia was conducted. The cohorts were each assigned a score of 0 to 5 based on the presence of clinical lesions, body condition, and activity level (0 = no lesions, 1 = lesions healing, 2 = mild ulceration with no affect on appetite or activity, 3 = moderate ulceration or crusting with mild affect on appetite or activity, 4 = extensive ulceration or crusting with noticeable weight loss and reduction in activity, 5 = active vesicles or severe loss of mucosal surfaces with marked reduction in weight and activity).

Descriptive analyses were performed at cow and farm levels. Overall, prevalence of VS-NJ and VS-IN were calculated as well as prevalence of each serotype by farm. For each farm, the percentage positive by date was organized and graphed. Also, the dates of seroconversion for each positive animal were analyzed. Finally, the frequency of each serotype by age for each farm was calculated. Sentinel herd sampling statistics and ELISA results for this study are presented in Tables 8.3 and 8.4.

TABLE 8.3   El Salvador Sentinel Dairy Farm Sampling Statistics

Farm number	Number of animals sampled	Median times each animal sampled	Seroprevalence (%)*		95% Confidence interval (%)	
			VSV-NJ	VSV-IN	VSV-NJ	VSV-IN
1	131	4	56	37[†]	47 to 65	29 to 46
2	102	4	11	16	5 to 17	9 to 24
3	167	3	2	9[†]	.03 to 4	4 to 14
4	140	4	9	9	4 to 14	4 to 14
5	125	4	85	22[†]	79 to 91	15 to 30
6	50	4	70	18[†]	57 to 82	7 to 29
7	89	4	76	21[†]	67 to 85	12 to 30
8	94	4	81	45[†]	73 to 89	35 to 55
9	134	5	59	30[†]	50 to 68	22 to 38
10	107	4	53	10[†]	43 to 63	4 to 16
11	23	19	83	70	68 to 99	51 to 89
12	58	3	90	70[†]	82 to 98	58 to 82

*Apparent prevalence adjusted to true prevalence.

[†]$P < .05$ for χ^2 test for proportions comparing seroprevalence of VSV-NJ and VSV-IN for each sentinel farm.

Abbreviations: VSV-NJ, vesicular stomatitis virus–New Jersey; VSV-IN, vesicular stomatitis virus–Indiana.

TABLE 8.4   Enzyme-linked immunosorbent assay percent positive cohorts on El Salvador sentinel dairy farms by year and virus serotype.

Farm number	VSV-NJ (%)			VSV-IN (%)		
	1998	1999	2001	1998	1999	2001
1	0	48	70*	0.0	37	19[†]
2	0	9	0*	0	12	2[†]
3	0	4	1*	0	7	0[†]
4	0	5	4*	0	6	0[†]
5	65	54	70*	13	12	9
6	74	73	ND	26	35	ND
7	63	59	ND	22	1	ND[†]
8	67	85	81*	29	33	3[†]
9	25	23	39	4	8	5
10	21	33	7*	2	1	0
11	72	42	ND*	47	42	ND
12	80	87	93	32	40	13[†]
Total	28	32	33	9	16	5

* χ^2 test for proportions of VSV-NJ seropositive cohorts between years significant at $P < .01$.
[†] χ^2 test for proportions of VSV-IN seropositive cohorts between years significant at $P < .01$.
Abbreviations: VSV-NJ, vesicular stomatitis virus–New Jersey; VSV-IN, vesicular stomatitis virus–Indiana.

This sentinel project served a dual purpose. The epidemiology of VS had not been previously investigated in El Salvador. Peak time of transmission, potential vectors and reservoirs, and disease prevalence in general were unknown. The primary purpose of the design of this sentinel project was an attempt to investigate the ecology and epidemiology of VS in endemic areas of El Salvador and to compare this information with similar data collected in the sporadically epidemic regions of the United States. Second, monthly visits by veterinarians on operations that may not ordinarily have a veterinarian ever visit establishes a disease surveillance system for all diseases potentially affecting cattle and other livestock species present on the operation.

SENTINEL HERDS IN COLORADO AND NEW MEXICO

Vesicular stomatitis outbreaks in the United States are closely monitored by the USDA's Animal and Plant Health Inspection Service, Veterinary Services (APHIS-VS), and during the last three outbreaks (in 1995, 1997, and 1998), premises and animal information was maintained in a database. There are many individual premises that have been designated as positive during more than one outbreak, and a majority of positive premises primarily maintained horses and not cattle (McCluskey et al. 1999). The primary purpose of establishing sentinel research herds was to test the hypothesis that vesicular stomatitis viruses were present in the southwestern United States in nonoutbreak years; this was not to attempt to detect VS at a predetermined level or to conduct surveillance for other diseases or disease agents.

Only sentinel equine herds were selected because horses were more accessible on a routine sampling scheme and greater than 75%, 97%, and 98% of the positive premises were identified as equine operations in the 1995, 1997, and 1998 outbreaks, respectively. To improve the probability of detection of viral activity in the sentinel herds, herds that had been designated positive in at least one but preferably more than one of the last three outbreaks, had at least two horses, and were located in areas that had experienced extensive viral activity in one of the last three outbreaks were selected from outbreak databases (Figure 8.2). A total of 20 herds in Colorado and 20 herds in New Mexico were initially enlisted to participate. Once herds were selected from the outbreak databases, herd owners were contacted and their willingness to participate in a 3-year study was determined. Paste anthelmintics were offered during each visit for each horse in the study as an incentive to continue in the study. Quarterly visits were made to each sentinel premises in which between two and 20 sentinel horses were given examinations of the mouth, nasal cavity, feet, and external genitalia. In addition, blood samples were drawn by jugular venipuncture and swabs were collected from the oral cavity. Information about premises management practices, animal movement history, and other potential risk factors were collected by a standardized questionnaire at each visit.

All serum samples were tested by the competitive ELISA (cELISA) for antibody to both VSV serotypes. Samples positive by one or both cELISAs were tested by IgM capture ELISA, complement fixation tests, and serum neutralization tests for each serotype of the virus. Oral swab samples were frozen at $-70°C$ until the completion of serological testing.

Descriptive statistics include overall farm-level prevalence and incidence densities. Survival analysis was used to allow for inclusion of censored horses. A seroconversion was considered a "failure" in the survival analysis. Kaplan-Meier curves were generated for those premises with horses that seroconverted so that the mean survival time could be calculated. Mean survival time for each premises was used in a general linear model to evaluate management, environmental, and other factors associated with variations in survival times (McCluskey et al. 2002).

Methods of analysis of data from sentinel herd schemes are discussed in more detail in Chapters 5 and 6.

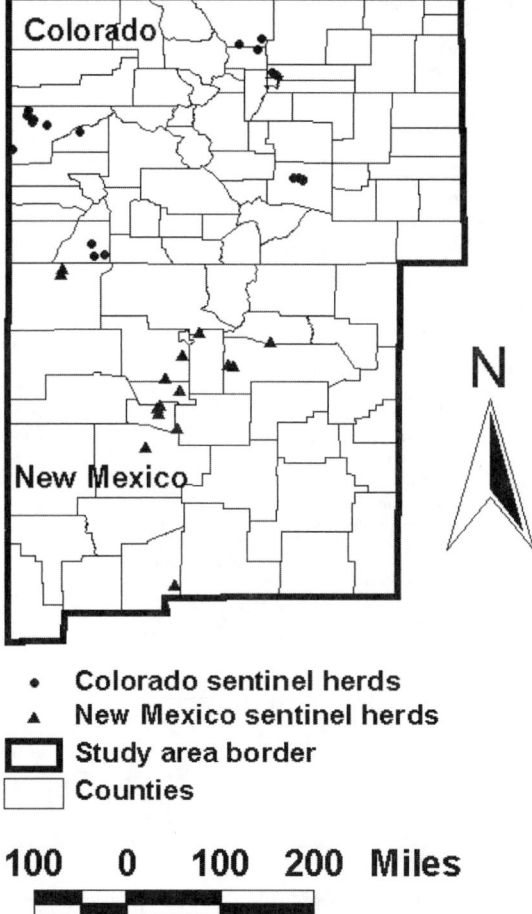

FIGURE 8.2   Distribution of vesicular stomatitis virus cases in Colorado from the last three outbreaks.

CONCLUSIONS

Sentinel herd surveillance can be an appropriate and economic alternative to more conventional methods of animal health surveillance. The key to success of any surveillance system is the establishment of goals before its development and implementation. Sentinel surveillance is no exception to this rule. The steps necessary in establishing sentinel herd surveillance are summarized in Figure 8.3. Effective application of sentinel herd surveillance can enhance the overall animal health monitoring and surveillance programs of any country, ultimately leading to healthier livestock and more financially competitive livestock industries.

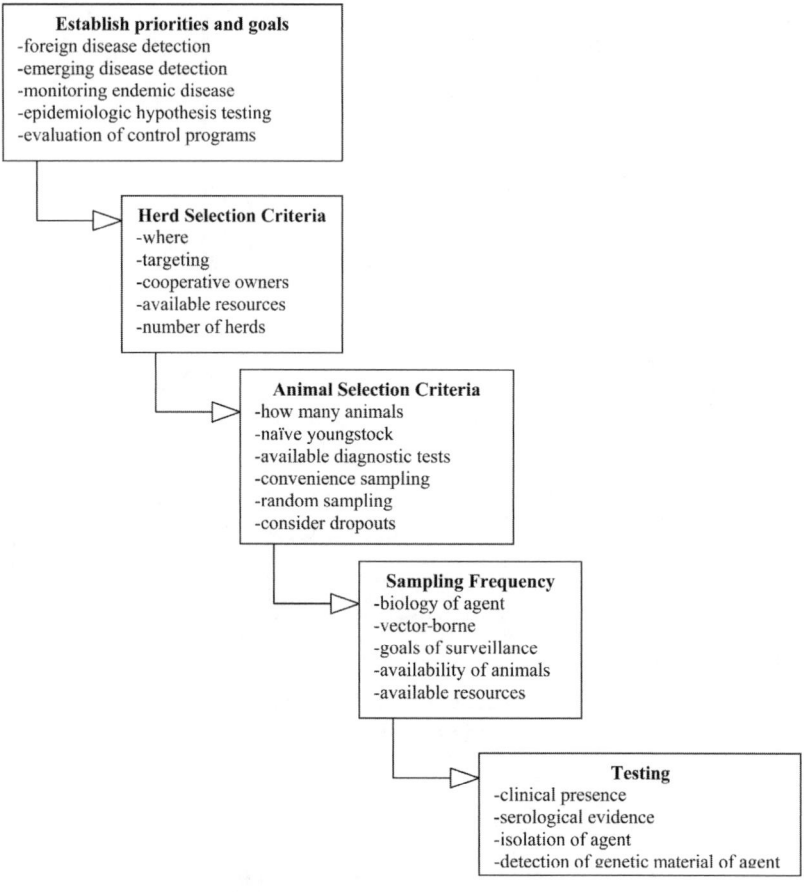

FIGURE 8.3   Considerations in establishing sentinel herd surveillance

BIBILOGRAPHY

Animal Health Australia. 2001. Animal health in Australia 2000. Australian Ministry of Agriculture, Canberra, Australia, p 29.

Cameron A.R., Baldock F.C. 1998. A new probability formula for surveys to substantiate freedom from disease. Prev Vet Med 34:1–17.

Kellar J. 1999. Sentinel herd applications in Canada. CAHnet Bull Summer 1999, ed. 3, Ontario, Canada.

McCluskey B.J., Hurd H.S., Mumford E.L. 1999. Review of the 1997 outbreak of vesicular stomatitis in the western United States. J Am Vet Med Assoc 215:1259–1262.

McCluskey B.J., Mumford E.L., Salman M.D., Traub-Dargatz, J.L. 2002. Use of sentinel herds to study the epidemiology of vesicular stomatitis in the State of Colorado. Ann N Y Acad Sci 969:205–209.

Parrish R.G., McDonnell S.M. 1994. Sources of routinely collected data for surveillance. In: Principles and practice of public health surveillance, S.M. Teutsch and R.E. Churchill (Eds.). Oxford University Press, New York, pp 45–51.

Thacker S.B., Choi K., Brachman P.S. 1983. The surveillance of infectious diseases. J Am Med Assoc 249:1181–1185.

Thrusfield M. 1995. Veterinary epidemiology, 2nd ed. Cambridge University Press, London, p 179.

Valleron A.J., Garnerin P. 1992. Computer networking as a tool for public health surveillance: The French experiment. Proceedings of the 1992 International Symposium in Public Health Surveillance. Morb Mort World Rep 41(suppl.):101–110.

Use of Animal Monitoring and Surveillance Systems When the Frequency of Health-Related Events Is Near Zero

M.G. Doherr,[1] L. Audigé,[2] M.D. Salman,[3] and I.A. Gardner[4]

INTRODUCTION

The objective of this chapter is to review the current monitoring and surveillance system (MOSS) approaches in situations when the frequency of health-related events, clinical disease, or measurable infection is rare. This includes the

[1]Division for Clinical Research, Department of Clinical Veterinary Medicine, University of Bern, Bremgartenstrasse 109a, CH-3001 Bern, Switzerland

[2]AO Clinical Investigation and Documentation, AO Center, Clavadelerstrasse, CH-7270 Davos Platz, Switzerland

[3]Animal Population Health Institute, College of Veterinary Medicine and Biomedical Sciences, Colorado State University, Ft. Collins, CO 80523–1681

[4]Department of Medicine and Epidemiology, School of Veterinary Medicine, University of California, Davis, California 95616

scenario of when the animal population in a given geographic region is approaching freedom from infection with given pathogen or from clinical disease.

Traditionally, animal populations are periodically or continuously monitored by stakeholders such as animal owners, livestock industries, or veterinary services for clinical disease or infection with a given pathogen that could potentially threaten animal or human health and well-being—that could hamper trade or reduce production and, therefore, revenue. Early detection and rapid intervention of infectious disease outbreaks has been of paramount importance in the control of classical swine fever (CSF), foot and mouth disease (FMD), rinderpest, and other diseases included in list A of the Office International des Epizooties (OIE; http://www.oie.int/eng/maladies/en_classification.htm).

The level of occurrence of some of these infectious diseases at the beginning of outbreak or at its end may be so low that they can be missed by conventional MOSS. Missing those rare events might prevent the implementation of control measures. This could result in larger, longer, or new outbreaks.

In recent years, the World Trade Organization (WTO)'s Agreement on the Application of Sanitary and Phytosanitary Measures (SPS) on plant and animal trade (1995) has specified the conditions under which trade in animals and animal products between countries could be legally restricted. One of the allowable conditions to restrict free trade is that the importing country can document that its animal population has a higher animal health status (regarding specific infectious or zoonotic diseases) than the potential trading partner, in which case the products from the exporting country pose an (unacceptable) health risk to the human or domestic animal population of the receiving country. This SPS agreement, together with OIE and other organizations such as European Commission (EC) attempts to categorize countries as high-prevalence (or "risk"), low-prevalence, or disease-free regions for specific diseases or pathogens, and the development of screening tests for a range of livestock diseases, has resulted in a demand for disease-free certifications. Countries no longer only have to monitor their animal populations for obvious outbreaks of exotic, or foreign animal diseases (FADs), but they also have to perform extensive surveys or ongoing surveillance activities (or both) to control or eradicate other (often endemic) livestock diseases and to document to others the disease status of their animal population. This documentation of status has frequently been extended from the absence of clinical disease to the absence of the infectious agent or, as in the case of monitoring for infectious bovine rhinotracheitis (IBR) in several European countries, to the absence of serologic reactors to specific infectious agents (no animals with positive antibody titer).

One difficulty is that the term "disease freedom" is used rather broadly. The situation of total absence of the infectious agent in all host species, all potential vectors, and the environment would mark one end of the "freedom" scale.

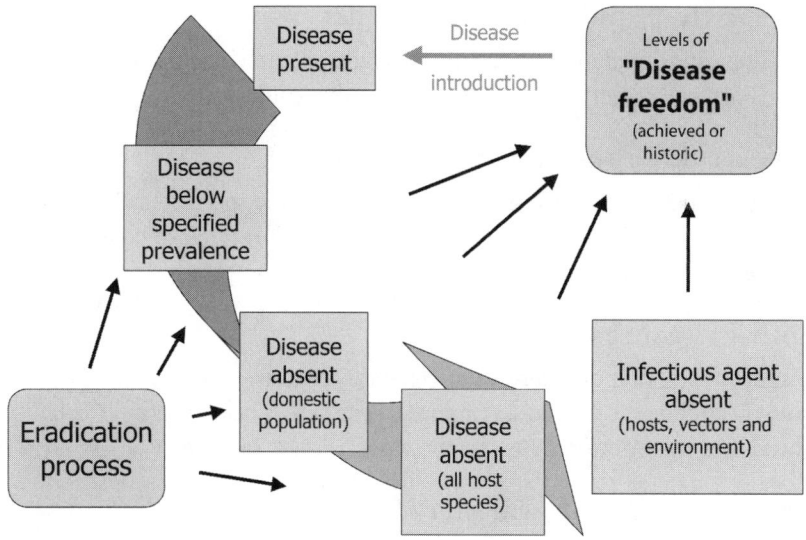

FIGURE 9.1   Levels of disease freedom in different host populations achieved historically or through targeted control measures (eradication process).

The presence of the infectious agent—or even clinical disease—at an "acceptable" level in the target species of interest or in another population such as wildlife hosts is at the other end of the freedom scale (Figure 9.1). Disease classification using MOSS approaches needs to be adapted to the type of health event (i.e., clinical disease, infectious agent, etc.), the current position of the individual countries or regions on a specific scale (Dufour and La Vieille 2000), and the purpose that health authorities want to achieve. Under these conditions, the total absence of pathogen may not be possible. In the context of this chapter, we will limit the discussion to examples of MOSS systems for events within livestock populations.

DEFINITIONS

For the purpose of this chapter, we will use the following terms as defined here.

Measurable Event

A measurable event is any event that can be detected with the diagnostic tests that are currently available. In the context of this chapter, this is limited to events such as clinical disease, presence of infectious agents in an animal, or evidence of exposure (such as antibodies) that can be measured with standard test systems.

Domestic Population of a Country

The domestic population of a country includes all individuals of a species that were born and raised and are maintained in that country.

Livestock Population

All individual animals from the common livestock species (such as cattle, sheep, goats, swine, and poultry) in a given (defined) region or country make up the livestock population.

Unit of Interest

The structural unit of interest for which the disease or infection status is assessed could be the individual (animal), pen, herd, flock, or farm or could be the higher organizational structures such as a region or country.

Freedom (Zero Prevalence/Incidence)

Freedom is defined as complete absence of an event from a defined population at a given point in time (prevalence) or for a period of time (incidence). Proof of true freedom, especially for dynamic events such as infectious diseases, theoretically requires a perfect measuring (test) system and the simultaneous examination of all units within the population.

Sample Prevalence (Or Incidence)

Prevalence (or incidence) of an event within a defined target population that was derived from a representative subset or sample of that population is termed sample prevalence. This estimate can be extrapolated to the target population from which the sample was drawn.

Prevalence or Incidence near Zero

The prevalence or incidence of measurable events in a given population (of units of interest) that has declined to levels that are only detectable with very extensive surveys, and that result in negative survey results (perceived freedom, probable freedom) from routine MOSSs is described as prevalence (or incidence) near zero.

MONITORING METHODS WHEN THE PREVALENCE OF MEASURABLE EVENTS OR THE INCIDENCE OF NEW EVENTS APPROACHES ZERO

Within this section, the standard approaches that are used to assess low levels of disease occurrence approaching zero are presented. This includes ongoing monitoring and surveillance activities and cross-sectional (population) surveys. The use of historical data as evidence of disease freedom is presented in the section below.

GENERAL STATISTICAL CONSIDERATIONS OF SAMPLING APPROACHES

The general statistical considerations for sampling approaches are described in Chapter 5. In cases in which the prevalence of interest in a population is approaching zero, sample sizes required to detect such low prevalence levels quickly increase toward the total population size.

An additional component of complexity is the way the disease clusters within the population. Infectious diseases that are spread by animal contact can be rare at the herd level (only very few herds infected) but have prevalences exceeding 50% in infected herds. IBR is an example in which countries such as Switzerland are considered to be disease-free at the herd level (Audigé et al. 2001; Stärk 1996). This is documented annually by surveys in which a sufficient randomly selected number of herds are tested to document that the prevalence of affected herds does not exceed a predetermined level, such as 0.1%. The survey makes use of the fact that the within-herd prevalence is expected to be high, and hence, IBR-infected herds are detected with high confidence once a sufficient number of animals from those herds are tested. This approach is described in more detail in Chapter 5.

A contrasting example is that of bovine spongiform encephalopathy (BSE), where exposure took place through widely distributed feed components. Especially in the countries with lower case frequencies, only one cattle per affected farm was diagnosed with the disease. As a consequence, sampling strategies and sample sizes need to be adapted to the low within-herd prevalence of detectable cases. This is one of the reasons why targeted BSE MOSS is not herd-based but mainly relies on the examination of all high-risk animals that leave the population.

HISTORICAL DISEASE FREEDOM

Some countries have maintained a long history of freedom from many diseases in lists A and B of the OIE. The ability to maintain this free status has in part been attributable to geographic isolation combined with prohibition of quarantine restrictions applied to imported animals and animal products. Even when all areas of a country have not been able to achieve disease-free status, some zones or states within a country have been able to achieve disease-free status through regulated animal movements and appropriate surveillance methods.

The OIE has developed standards for declaring freedom from two list A diseases: rinderpest and contagious bovine pleuropneumonia. However, such standards have not been developed for the other 13 list A diseases, any list B diseases (including bovine brucellosis and porcine reproductive and respiratory syndrome virus [PRRS]), or for other economically important livestock diseases such as Johne's disease (JD, *Mycobacterium paratuberculosis*). Hence, individual countries, regions, and zones typically decide on what surveillance or survey data are necessary to substantiate their claims of disease freedom. This evidence is usually presented to trading partners, who consider it along with other factors such as the quality of veterinary services.

The approaches to disease surveillance and the necessary evidence to document disease freedom can differ if a country has historically been free of disease compared with the scenario when a disease is being eradicated and prevalence is approaching zero. In the latter case, there are at least four factors that might modify the choice of surveillance and survey methods:

1. Use of vaccination during an eradication program complicates interpretation of test results because few diagnostic tests can differentiate vaccinated noninfected animals from naturally infected animals.
2. Modifications to surveillance programs are often needed as prevalence (proportion of infected herds and within-herd prevalence in infected herds) changes. For example, more specific diagnostic tests or testing strategies are often used to avoid unacceptably high false-positive rates in the final stages of an eradication campaign (Salman 1998).
3. More rigorous designs and more extensive data often are necessary to initially establish rather than maintain disease-free status. Typically, larger sample sizes (numbers of herds and numbers of animals within a herd) might be needed to establish freedom, but fewer samples might be necessary during subsequent testing (Audigé et al. 1999).
4. Use of risk-based sampling of high-risk groups can be more easily implemented when there is experience with patterns of disease in a country. These risk groups might be geographically defined; for example, along border areas or in generally animal-dense areas. For example, targeted sampling for exotic viral diseases in Denmark is done along the Danish-German border, for example, Southern Jutland, where previously, a high risk of airborne transmission of pseudorabies (Aujeszky's disease) virus has been demonstrated (Stärk et al. 2000). Also, the main target of an active MOSS for BSE should be the population of adult sick (or dead) cattle that leave the population (emergency slaughter, fallen stock), as in these subpopulations, the prevalence of detectable cases is the highest (Doherr et al. 1999, 2001, 2002).

EXAMPLES

In the following sections, we consider four disease examples to demonstrate the variability in approach to surveillance and survey methods when countries have historically been disease free, compared with the scenario where the disease is being eradicated and prevalence is approaching zero. The first example is rinderpest, for which the pathway to disease freedom has been defined by OIE. The second example is brucellosis in the United States, for which political and economic ramifications will to a large extent determine choice of long-term surveillance methods. Examples three (PRRS [Porcine Respiratory and Reproductive Syndrome]) and four (JD [Johne's Disease]) show how consideration of disease epidemiology, accuracy of available tests, and identification of high-risk groups can be incorporated into the design of surveillance programs and surveys to document disease freedom at a country and state level, respectively.

WORLDWIDE ERADICATION OF RINDERPEST

Global eradication of rinderpest is targeted for 2010, and much of the cattle-producing world is designated as free or provisionally free of infection (www.oie.int). Current foci of rinderpest exist in eastern Africa and west and south Asia. However, in many African and Asian countries, infection has been successfully eradicated through strategic use of vaccination.

The OIE has defined a 4-year pathway for countries to achieve the target of disease freedom (James 1998). In brief, if no rinderpest has been detected for at least 2 years, the risk of reintroduction through animal movements is minimized, and vaccination is stopped, a country may declare provisional freedom from infection. If no seropositive cases are identified via serological surveillance in the country in the following 2 years, the country may be declared totally free of rinderpest infection. After the cessation of vaccination, the potential consequences of nondetected infection become more serious as the proportion of nonvaccinated susceptible animals increases. However, epidemiologic surveillance ensures that there is concomitant reduction in the risk that infection could persist, and if detected, it ensures that no major epidemic would result.

Sampling and testing procedures for rinderpest must be designed to give 95% confidence annually of detecting seropositive animals in any relevant age group if any were present in the 1% of the herds or other sampling units. Cattle and other susceptible domestic animals must be included in the serologic screening. On the basis of lack of evidence of virus activity and subject to the review of the serologic surveillance program and other requirements, the OIE might declare freedom from rinderpest infection.

For countries historically free of rinderpest, restriction on importation of ruminants from infected or provisionally disase-free countries, and an effective surveillance program that includes investigation of suspected epidemics, might be adequate evidence of continued freedom.

BRUCELLOSIS ERADICATION IN THE UNITED STATES

The United States has about 33 million beef cattle and about 9 million dairy cattle. Brucellosis is nearly eradicated from cattle populations: As of January 2002, there was only one known infected herd present in the population. An important unanswered question is how best to maintain surveillance of the cattle population to ensure early detection and eradication of infection and subsequent verification of disease freedom. There are a number of surveillance and survey options that are being considered (Salman 1998), each with different cost and political acceptability and ease of implementation.

The main choices available include use of the MCI (market cattle identification) program in slaughtered cattle with traceback of test-positive animals to their herds of origin with follow-up testing, a combination of the MCI program with annual serologic testing of a scientifically based sample of live cattle, this combination with the modification that sampling of live cattle is done every 3 years, serologic testing of a scientifically based sample of live cattle every 3 years but no MCI program, and collection of milk and lymph nodes from a scientifically based sample of live cattle.

The advantages and disadvantages of these choices are described in detail elsewhere (Salman 1998). However, they highlight the complexity in choosing the optimal program.

PRRS IN AUSTRALIA

PRRS virus was first detected in Europe in 1990, and over the next decade spread to most major swine-producing countries worldwide. Through rigorous import restrictions, Australia has maintained its freedom from the virus. Between 1995 and 1997, four investigations of PRRS-like disease were done, and all were negative. In 1997, a national survey of finisher pigs (approximately 6 months old) was done to document freedom (Garner et al. 1997). The survey was designed to provide 99% confidence of detecting at least one infected pig herd, assuming that at least 25% of finisher pigs in an infected herd had antibodies to the virus. Principles of herd-level sensitivity and specificity were considered in the survey design. During February 1996, 163 herds were sampled and 875 sera tested by a commercial PRRS enzyme-linked immunosorbent assay (ELISA). All major swine-producing areas were represented. Seven samples were ELISA-positive (serum-to-positive ratio of > 0.4), but all were found subsequently to be negative by indirect fluorescent antibody test. The combination of the lack of detection of virus in suspected field outbreaks and the negative survey results were considered adequate to document country-level freedom.

JD IN CATTLE IN WESTERN AUSTRALIA

Demonstration of freedom from a chronic infectious disease such as JD is problematic because of the long incubation period, the typically low to moderate within-herd prevalence, and the low sensitivity of available diagnostic tests.

JD in cattle is commonly found in cattle herds in eastern Australian states, but Western Australia has had no evidence on infection in its cattle herds, except for five imported infected cattle detected between 1980 and 1997 (Ellis et al. 1998). In all cases, infection was successfully eradicated by depopulation of cattle and verified by subsequent monitoring.

Between 1989 and 1993, an extensive survey of cattle herds including high-risk groups was done. The following herds were tested (Ellis et al. 1998):

1. Five herds that had previously had cases of Johne's disease.
2. Nine herds that had imported cattle from interstate herds that subsequently had, or were suspected of having, JD.
3. Forty-four herds that had imported dairy cattle from Australian states where JD typically occurs.
4. One hundred two herds that had imported at least five groups of beef cattle from Australian states with endemic JD in beef cattle and that were located in regions of southern Western Australia with higher rainfall (> 500 mm per annum).

Of tested cattle, 7,233 were negative, and 59 were ELISA positive. Ninety-seven herds gave all negative results, and the positive results were distributed over 30 herds. All fecal samples from cattle with positive initial ELISA tests were negative on fecal culture for *M. avium paratuberculosis*. The negative results in the survey taken alone may not be sufficient to gain enough confidence in the absence of JD, but combined with the long history of freedom in nonimported cattle and strict movement and import requirements, the overall information was considered adequate evidence by veterinary authorities of state-level freedom from JD.

ARE NEW MONITORING APPROACHES NEEDED?

In the previous sections, we have presented the most common MOSSs used to assess the disease status of a population once the prevalence is low. The objective of a MOSS is to provide sufficient information to substantiate a claim of disease freedom or to estimate the low but nonzero prevalence. However, the approaches taken may differ considerably. It remains a major challenge to provide comparable (between time and animal populations) estimates of prevalence or the probability of disease freedom. Once a reliable (and internationally accepted) methodology has been developed that allows us to critically evaluate MOSS approaches in place and that derives probabilities of disease freedom or estimates of low disease frequencies by weighing and pooling MOSS data from different sources, a reliable comparison of such data between populations might become possible.

The validity of all MOSS activities is most often questioned when the outcome is negative; that is, when no cases were reported or detected by the system. Nevertheless, based on this negative finding, the investigators or veterinary authorities often simply conclude that the target population is free of the event under scrutiny. Because surveillance for rare health-related events and the designation of freedom from infection have become increasingly important for veterinary authorities, researchers have started to investigate such methods to assess especially the overall diagnostic validity of MOSS activities (e.g., from baseline surveillance or targeted screening) and thus better interpret their results. Also, new approaches are under development to combine surveillance data from several sources into an overall probability estimate of disease freedom for a given country or region. Targeted surveys, as previously described, have been used for a range of diseases to compare the outcome with the data from the parallel operating baseline MOSS to assess the respective levels of case ascertainment and case reporting. Introducing a targeted screening component can, in addition to identifying additional cases of disease, increase the disease awareness and provide an incentive for reporting clinical suspect cases.

Depending on the disease, the country (region) of interest, and the diagnostic tests available, strategies to combine baseline MOSSs with targeted screening of selected populations have now been successfully implemented. A combination of baseline monitoring (for new clinical cases) and targeted screening (for sero-positive animals) has been used to determine the end of contagious disease outbreaks of CSF and FMD in previously disease-free countries.

One major area for further development is the issue of survey design. Sampling strategies and sample sizes need to be adjusted for the demography of the target population, the disease of interest, and the diagnostic test characteristics. New manuals and software tools have been made available for this purpose (Cameron 1999). When good estimates of the population structure, individual animal diagnostic test characteristics, sampling scheme, and epidemiology of the disease (condition) of interest are available, simulation models can be constructed to assess the feasibility of a given targeted survey even before it is done or to assist in the interpretation of survey results (Audigé and Beckett 1999;

Audigé et al. 1999, 2000, 2001). Simulation modeling is described in detail in Chapter 10.

Recently published international recommendations, or requirements, for disease surveillance and control typically require an integrated approach that includes an assessment of the risk factors for disease presence, mandatory reporting of clinical suspects, and targeted screening activities to supplement the results, especially those from the passive type of MOSS. Examples are the rinderpest surveillance and control guidelines (International Atomic Energy Agency [IAEA] 1994; OIE 1998, 2000a) and contagious bovine pleuropneumonia (OIE 2000b), and the requirements or recommendations for BSE and scrapie surveillance (European Commission 1999; OIE 2000c–2000e). New analytic methods are currently under development to analyze data from complex MOSS approaches. In an attempt to combine data from a range of (parallel or serial) surveillance sources, Hueston and Yoe (2000) proposed the use of probabilistic scenario analysis and event trees to identify and assess the major pathways by which disease can be detected. They conclude that the approach is well suited to evaluate and rank the relative effectiveness of a set of approaches for MOSS.

CONCLUSION

In conclusion, the existing tools for monitoring and surveillance all have their limitations once the events of interest become rare. Users of those methods and recipients of data from such approaches should be aware of those limitations and of the validity of the results produced. New approaches could include the individual development of MOSS strategies that are disease specific and population specific. Also, new methods to combine MOSS data from various sources need to be developed and evaluated with real-time data. BSE and other diseases for which large, ongoing MOSS activities employ different strategies might provide a good data source for such method development.

BIBLIOGRAPHY

Audigé, L., Beckett, S. 1999. A quantitative assessment of the validity of animal-health surveys using stochastic modelling. Prev Vet Med 38:259–276.

Audigé L.M., Doherr M.G., Hauser R., Wagner B., Salman M. 2000. A stochastic simulation model for the planning and quantitative assessment of herd-level testing scheme and surveys. Proceedings of the International Society for Veterinary Epidemiology and Economics, 6-11August 2000, Breckenridge, CO.

Audigé L., Doherr M.G., Hauser R., Salman M.D. 2001. Stochastic modelling as a tool for planning animal-health surveys and interpreting screening-test results. Prev Vet Med 49:1–17.

Audigé L., Doherr M.G., Salman M. 1999. A quantitative approach in declaring a country free of a disease. Proceedings of the Society for Veterinary Epidemiology and Preventive Medicine, 24–26 March 1999, University of Bristol, pp. 78–87.

Cameron A. 1999. Survey toolbox for livestock diseases—A practical manual and software package for active surveillance in developing countries. Australian Center for International Agricultural Research Monograph no. 54, pp 330.

Doherr M.G., Heim D., Fatzer R., Cohen C.H., Vandevelde M., Zurbriggen A. 2001. Targeted screening of high-risk cattle populations for BSE to augment mandatory reporting of clinical suspects. Prev Vet Med 51:3–16.

Doherr M.G., Hett A.R., Cohen C.H., Fatzer R., Rüfenacht J., Zurbriggen A., Heim D. 2002. Trends in prevalence of BSE in Switzerland based on fallen stock and slaughter surveillance. Vet Rec 150:347–348.

Doherr M.G., Oesch B., Moser B., Vandevelde M., Heim D. 1999. Targeted surveillance for bovine spongiform encephalopathy (BSE). Vet Rec 145:672–675.

Dufour B., La Vieille S. 2000. Epidemiological surveillance of infectious diseases in France. Vet Res 31:169–185.

Ellis T.M., Norris R.T., Martin P.A.J., Casey R.H., Hawkins C.D. 1998. Evidence of freedom from Johne's disease in cattle and goats in Western Australia. Aust Vet J 76:630–633.

European Commission. 1999. Surveillance of TSEs in sheep and goat in relation to the risk of infection with bovine spongiform encephalopathy agent and related actions to be taken at EU level. Actions to be taken on the basis of (1) the September 1998 SSC Opinion on the risk of infection of sheep and goats with the BSE agent and (2) the April 1999 SEAC Subgroup report on research and surveillance for TSEs in sheep. Opinion of the Scientific Steering Committee, Consumer Health Protection, European Commission, adopted at the SSC meeting of 27–28 May 1999.

Garner M.G., Gleeson L.J., Holyoake P.K., Cannon R.M., Doughty W.J. 1997. A national serological survey to verify Australia's freedom from porcine reproductive and respiratory syndrome. Aust Vet J 75:596–600.

Hueston W.D., Yoe C.E. 2000. Estimating the overall power of complex surveillance systems. Proceeding abstract 393, Ninth Meeting of the International Society of Veterinary Epidemiology and Economics. 6–12 August 2000, Breckenridge, CO.

International Atomic Energy Agency. 1994. Recommended procedures for disease and serological surveillance as part of the Global Rinderpest Eradication Programme. IAEA TECDOC 747, International Atomic Energy Agency, Vienna, Austria.

Office International des Epizooties. 1998. Guide to epidemiological surveillance for rinderpest. Rev Sci Technique 17:796–824.

Office International des Epizooties. 2000a. Recommended standard for epidemiological surveillance systems for Rinderpest. Office International des Epizooties, International Animal Health Code Part 3, Section 3.8, Appendix 3.8.1.

Office International des Epizooties. 2000b. Recommended standard for epidemiological surveillance systems for Contagious Bovine Pleuropneumonia. Office International des Epizooties, International Animal Health Code Part 3, Section 3.8, Appendix 3.8.2.

Office International des Epizooties. 2000c. Surveillance and monitoring of animal health. Office International des Epizooties, International Animal Health Code Part 1, Section 1.3, Chapter 1.3.5.

Office International des Epizooties. 2000d. Surveillance and monitoring systems for Bovine Spongiform Encephalopathy. Office International des Epizooties, International Animal Health Code Part 3, Section 3.8, Appendix 3.8.3.

Office International des Epizooties. 2000e. Bovine Spongiform Encephalopathy. Office International des Epizooties, International Animal Health Code Part 2, Section 2.3, Chapter 2.3.13.

Salman M. 1998. A monitoring system for program diseases that are reaching the level of eradication. Proc US Anim Health Assoc 1998:64–70.

Stärk K.D., Mortensen S., Olsen A.M., Barfod K., Bøtner A., Lavritsen D.T., Strandbygård B. (2000) Designing serological surveillance programmes to document freedom from disease with special reference to exotic viral diseases of pigs in Denmark. Rev Sci tech Off int Epiz 19(3):715–724.

Stärk K.D. 1996. Animal health monitoring and surveillance in Switzerland. Aust Vet J 73:96–97.

Use of Simulation Models in Surveillance and Monitoring Systems

L. Audigé,[1] M.G. Doherr,[2] and B. Wagner[3]

INTRODUCTION

Veterinary epidemiologists have extensively used different modeling techniques to better understand and predict disease processes within animal populations. This chapter focuses on a category of models called simulation models. Details on the different categories of models can be found in Martin et al. (1987), Hurd and Kaneene (1993), and Thrusfield (1995). Hurd and Kaneene (1993) distinguished simulation models as associative or process models, as illustrated in Figure 10.1. Modelers might be interested in risk factor or associative models to quantify etiologic associations between some risk factors and the occurrence of

[1]AO Clinical Investigation and Documentation, AO Center, Clavadelerstrasse, CH-7270 Davos Platz, Switzerland

[2]Division for Clinical Research, Department of Clinical Veterinary Medicine, University of Bern, Bremgartenstrasse 109a, CH-3012 Bern, Switzerland

[3]USDA:APHIS:VS:CEAH, Mail Stop #2E7, 2150 Centre Avenue, Building B, Fort Collins, CO 80526–8117

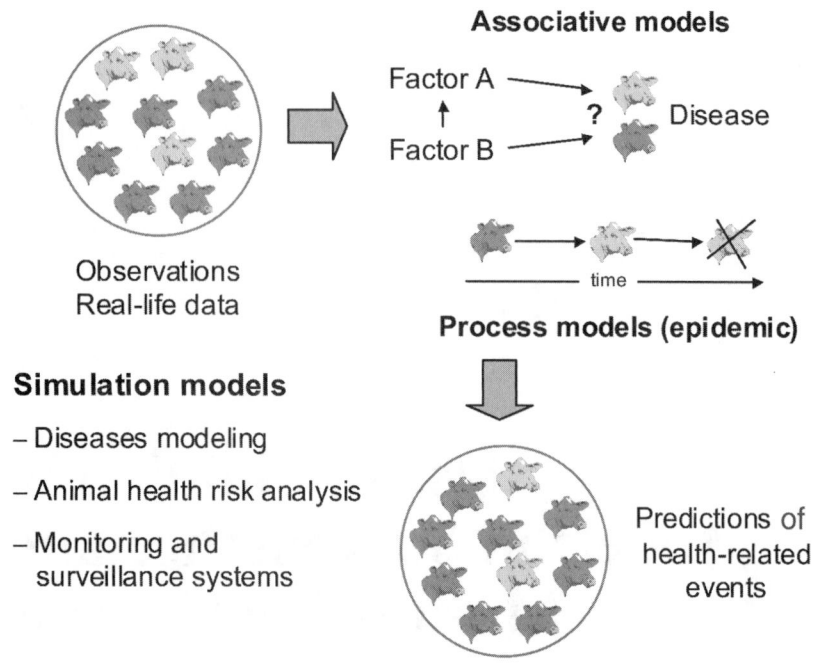

FIGURE 10.1   Different types of models used in veterinary epidemiology.

a disease and would use a logistic regression model to achieve this objective. As an alternative, process or transition models are constructed in an attempt to explain a disease process through time in a dynamic population. These models are often used to simulate plausible real-life scenarios (e.g., the presence and spread of an infection in an animal population) to make predictions regarding the most likely health-related outcomes in a population.

Simulation models have been used in veterinary science to increase understanding of disease epidemics and to investigate control strategies, such as with bovine spongiform encephalopathy (BSE; Anderson et al. 1996) and foot and mouth disease (FMD; Keeling et al. 2001; Morris et al. 2001). More recently, simulation models have been increasingly used for risk analysis in animal health (Vose 1996, 1997) following the requirements of the World Trade Organization (WTO) regarding trade of animals and animal products (WTO 1995; Carpenter et al. 1998; Zepeda et al. 2001). The New Zealand Ministry of Agriculture and Fisheries (MAF) has published such risk analysis reports on its Web site (MAF 2002). The ultimate goal of these simulation models was to support the decision-making process for future disease prevention and control strategies by estimating the probability of plausible real-world scenarios.

Animal-health decisions for disease control programs, animal trade, or disease-freedom certification rely on accurate, scientifically based knowledge of the health status of animals within a targeted animal population. The underlying question is to what extent or magnitude (incidence/prevalence level) does the disease actually occur in the population. The implementation of appropriate animal-health monitoring and surveillance systems (MOSSs) is required to develop information to address this question. This chapter presents the use of simulation modeling in MOSS activities and highlights areas for potential development.

DETERMINISTIC VERSUS STOCHASTIC SIMULATION

Simulation modeling can be deterministic or stochastic. In a deterministic model, input parameters are specified as point estimates, which could be any fixed value such as minimum, mean, or maximum values. Deterministic simulation models are relatively easy to implement and each calculation would reflect the outcome of one possible scenario. The ability to draw conclusions from deterministic models, however, is limited. This is because of the fact that it does not capture the inherent uncertainty of input parameters (as probability distributions) on model outcomes. In addition, in most situations, as in MOSS activities, realistic scenarios are too numerous and complex to compute, given the variation of influencing parameters and possible inter-relationships between them. In such complex situations, a deterministic approach can be cumbersome or very difficult to conduct.

The term "stochastic" refers to a probabilistic process that incorporates some element of randomness. Point estimates are replaced by probability distributions that are sampled by a random process (Moore 1996; Rugen and Callahan 1996). These distributions represent the variation of the input parameters attributed to both true biologic variability and uncertainty. Uncertainty relates to imperfect knowledge about the parameters (Thompson and Graham 1986). A commonly used process for implementing stochastic simulations is the Monte Carlo sampling procedure, whereas another common procedure is Latin Hypercube sampling (Loh 1996). In Monte Carlo simulation modeling, input values are randomly sampled at each run (repetition or iteration) from predefined probability distributions for each of the random factors within the model. Each iteration produces one outcome, as in the deterministic approach, but the outcome is not static because the input variables are no longer fixed. Each outcome from all the iterations is combined to produce a distribution of outcomes that represents the variability and uncertainty in the input variables. The outcome distribution is presented usually in the form of a probability density function or cumulative density function (Moore 1996).

ISSUES TO BE CONSIDERED IN SIMULATION MODELING FOR MOSS

There is increased recognition among veterinary epidemiologists that surveys should be tailored according to targeted animal populations, type of infections, current infection status, and surveillance objectives (Dufour and Audigé 1997; Doherr and Audigé 2001). Major issues in the survey design that received considerable attention over the last decade in the veterinary epidemiologic literature are those of clustering of infection within herds, the need for aggregate testing accounting for the level of clustering, and the uncertainty in the screening test(s) characteristics (Wagner and Salman 2000).

Traditionally, the planning of herd-level testing schemes and surveys, in particular, sample size calculations, has relied on tables published by Cannon and Roe (1982; see Chapter 4). Their sample size calculations are based on several assumptions that are almost never met in reality and, under certain circumstances, could yield estimates with much lower confidence than expected. For instance, the calculation assumes a perfect animal-level screening test; that is, the test sensitivity and specificity are both 100%. Some tests, such as serologic tests for Johne's disease (Dargatz et al. 2001), however, are far from perfection and, thus, there is a need to account for this imperfection. Furthermore, the sample size calculation process applies for single homogeneous populations with available sampling frames. In reality, animals occur in clusters in which the cluster-level prevalence of infection likely varies. A more realistic and flexible approach, which accounts for the epidemiology of targeted infections and the variability of within-herd prevalence, was needed.

USE OF STOCHASTIC MODELING IN MOSS ACTIVITIES

Salman and Christensen set some conceptual definitions regarding various health statuses in the previous chapters (Chapters 1 and 2). Traditionally, surveys were planned either to estimate prevalence if investigators knew the infection occurred or, as a special case of estimation, to detect infection. The detection approach is more often encountered when the infection prevalence approaches zero. We propose to revise this concept and consider that investigators should be able to provide two results when their survey is completed. First, they need to state the confidence (given as probabilities) with regard to any of the several "freedom" statuses presented in Chapters 1 and 5, such as the absence of antibody-positive animals in a given population. Second, they need to provide an estimate of the prevalence, if the health event occurred. We will highlight the benefit of simulation modeling in deriving these two results. The design is important for both appropriate herd-level testing scheme and survey, so we address this issue first.

ASSESSMENT OF HERD-LEVEL TESTING SCHEMES AND SURVEY CHARACTERISTICS

Several important issues in herd-level testing were developed in the early 1990s. Martin et al. (1992) focused on the effect of imperfect tests. They introduced the concept of allowing the number of test-positive animals needed to declare a herd as infected to exceed one animal, to account for the occurrence of false-positive tests. This was followed by theoretical considerations over the effect of infection clustering (Donald 1993; Donald et al. 1994). Cameron and Baldock (1998a, 1998b) made an important contribution with the development of the program, FreeCalc, now included in the Survey Toolbox package (Cameron 2002), to help investigators plan and interpret surveys aimed at substantiating freedom from infection. Input parameters, however, still are specified as single values. Recently, Cannon (2001) proposed simplifications for sample size calculations given a poorly sensitive but 100% specific test. Earlier, Carpenter and Gardner (1996) used a simulation model to evaluate the expected herd-level sensitivities and predictive values, but herd size, sample size, and animal test characteristics were specified as single values. Jordan and McEwen (1998) introduced the use of stochastic modeling to account for the variability of parameters influencing herd-level testing, which is a more complex but perhaps more realistic approach.

In this section, we present a methodological approach to quantitatively assess the validity of two-stage animal health surveys while taking into account several influencing factors (Audigé and Beckett 1999; Audigé et al. 2001). The premise for this approach is that a herd-level sampling scheme is essentially a diagnostic test for identifying truly infected herds. Similarly, a survey is considered a diagnostic system aimed at identifying the infection in the targeted population, and thus, its validity (sensitivity and specificity) can be quantitatively assessed.

Overview of the Model Structure

The evaluation process involves Monte Carlo simulation. The structure of the model is graphically presented in Figure 10.2. In the first part of the model, the herd-level sensitivity and specificity are derived from two probability distributions for the number of animal-level positive tests expected from noninfected and infected herds, respectively. Input variables were the distribution of herd sizes in the target population, the number or proportion of animals sampled in tested herds, the distribution of infection prevalence within infected herds, the animal-level test sensitivity and specificity (or combined test characteristics if more than one test was used), and the cut-off proportion or number of test-positive animal samples over which tested herds would be classified as positive.

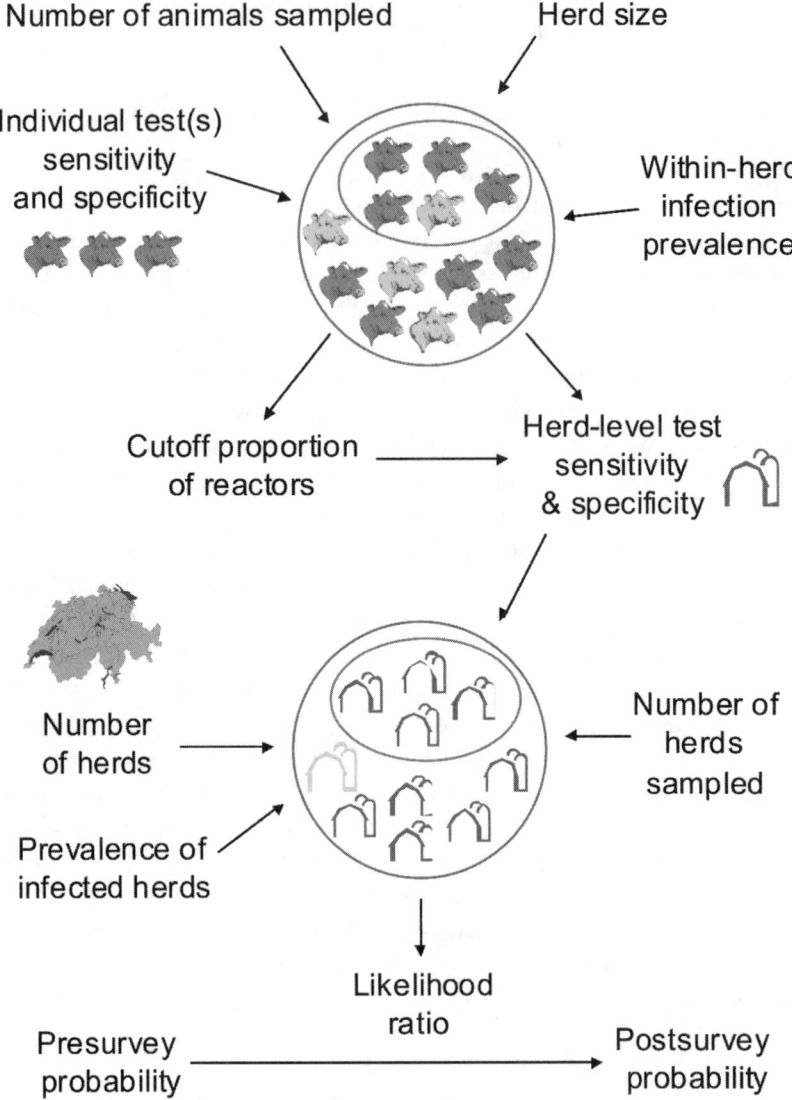

FIGURE 10.2   Model structure for quantitative assessment of herd-level sampling scheme and survey characteristics. The likelihood ratio (LR) was defined as the ratio of the probability of observing a specific survey result in the absence of the infection (true freedom) to the probability of observing the same result in the presence of the infection at a predefined herd prevalence.

The model allows for the variation of the proportion of animals sampled within selected herds. This proportion might be defined as a function of the herd size. An important assumption is that animals are randomly selected among all targeted animals within herds. The herd size corresponds to the number of animals within herds that are the focus of inference (e.g., all cows >2 years of age). Dependencies between several model input parameters, such as between herd size and infection prevalence, can be taken into account.

According to various possible cut-off proportions of test-positive animal samples, herd-level test sensitivity and specificity varies, and their values can be plotted on a Receiver Operating Characteristics (ROC) curve (Greiner et al. 2000). This curve can help to identify the most appropriate cut-off value for the given sampling scheme and survey objectives (Figure 10.3). For disease situations, within-herd sample sizes and screening test(s) might be chosen so that the simulated probability distributions of the number of positive tests from infected and noninfected herds do not overlap. In such a case, the optimal cut-off is that for which the herd-level sensitivity and specificity are close or equal to 100%. A compromise must be made otherwise, depending on whether high confidence in herd-level positive or negative testing is required. For instance, if you chose a cut-off at the level of the simulated probability distribution for the noninfected herds, the herd-level specificity will be 100% and the positive predictive value (i.e., your confidence in a positive herd level test) will be 100%. In any case, for a low prevalence level, this cut-off proportion or number approaches zero when the combined animal-level test specificity approaches 100%.

In the second part of the model, probability distributions for the number of positive herds expected in a situation of freedom from infection and under various levels of herd prevalence (proportion of herds in the country that are infected) are simulated. These distributions serve to determine survey sensitivity and specificity values and respective ROC curves (Figure 10.3b). Influencing factors are the number of herds in the population, the prevalence of infected herds in the population that the survey should be able to detect (threshold prevalence), the number of herds sampled, and the herd-level test sensitivity and specificity. The sample of herds is considered a random (thus representative) sample of the population of herds in the country or region. In addition to the survey characteristics, likelihood ratios are calculated to assist in the interpretation of actual (real-life) survey outcomes (Audigé et al. 2001).

Examples

Porcine Reproductive and Respiratory Syndrome

The model was developed specifically to assess the value of a slaughter survey aimed at substantiating freedom from porcine reproductive and respiratory syndrome (PRRS) in Switzerland (Canon et al. 1998). Blood samples were collected from fattened pigs at two slaughterhouses. Five samples per herd from a total of 108 herds were sampled over a period of 5 days and tested using an indirect enzyme-linked immunosorbent assay (ELISA). The contagious nature of the infection was important to consider; it was assumed that the prevalence

a) Herd-level test

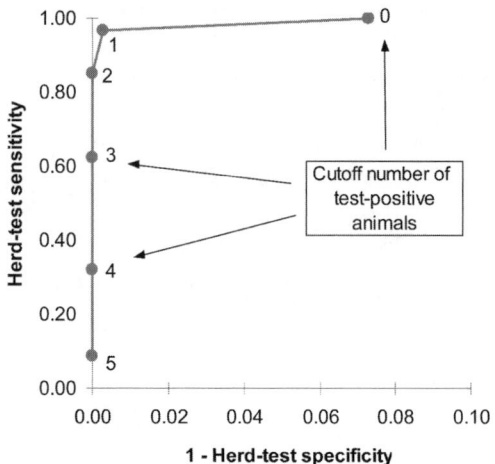

b) Survey

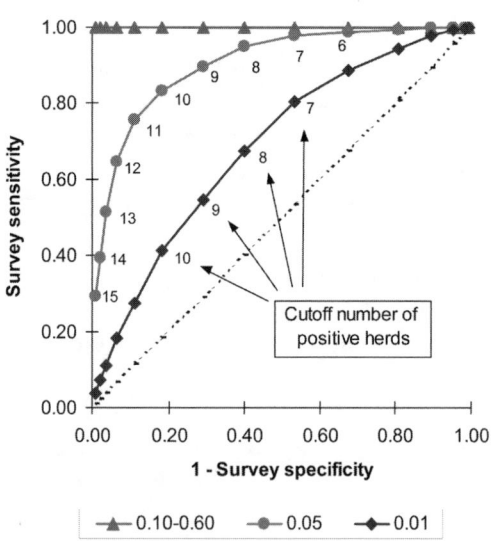

FIGURE 10.3   Output receiver operating characteristic curve of herd-level screening test and survey for seropositivity against Porcine Reproductive and Respiratory Syndrome virus in Switzerland. These figures are reproduced with permission from Elsevier (Audigé and Beckett 1999). (a) Five pigs were sampled per herd and tested by enzyme-linked immunosorbent assay; (b) 108 herds were sampled at slaughter and tested using the herd-level test presented in (a).

of infection most likely would be 60% in slaughtered pigs from infected herds, with a minimum of 10% and a maximum of 100% (within-herd prevalence), and that the herd prevalence would be over 10% (most likely 40% and maximum 60%), as observed in infected countries (Meredith 1995). From the herd-level test ROC curve shown in Figure 10.3a, it was decided to classify a herd as positive when at least one pig was tested positive (i.e., at least 20% of five samples).

Results from the simulation showed that the survey was highly sensitive and specific. It was determined to be almost impossible to observe the actual survey result (zero reactors) if PRRS occurred in the country at the time of sample collection at herd prevalence consistent with an endemic status (such as 10% or higher; Figure 10.3b). This model, thus, was useful in that it gave investigators confidence that the planned survey was large enough for its intended purpose.

This approach has the additional advantage of forcing investigators to critically review the evidence regarding information they had available for designing the survey; specifically, the distributions of model parameters. For instance, there was some discussion that the specificity of the ELISA used to test for PRRS antibodies might be higher than that stated by its developers. When testing results from a representative sample of a disease-free population are available (e.g., in previous negative survey results), the number of animals tested and false-positive test results can be used to define a distribution for the animal test specificity, using a beta distribution (see Audigé et al. 2001). The choice of the herd prevalence was justified given that the infection with PRRS viruses would spread rapidly between pig herds after introduction in an infection-free country. By considering various low herd prevalences nevertheless, an investigator can assess the ability of the survey to identify the infection at the start of an epidemic (i.e., shortly after its introduction). For example, the PRRS survey design presented above was inadequate to screen a population with a 1% herd-level prevalence (Audigé and Beckett 1999); for this threshold prevalence and the given survey design, the combined survey SE and survey SP were barely higher than 50%.

Newcastle Disease

The same modeling approach was used to assess a survey to investigate whether infection with low-pathogenic strains of Newcastle disease (ND) viruses occurred in laying hen flocks in Switzerland (Gohm et al. 1999). ND is a highly contagious viral disease of birds, particularly domestic poultry. At the time of the survey, Switzerland was officially declared free from ND as defined by the Office International des Epizooties (OIE), but no survey was routinely conducted on flocks.

Thirty blood samples from each of 260 commercial laying-hen flocks were collected in a central poultry slaughterhouse. Sera were screened for ND viral antibodies with an ELISA. We applied the model to help interpret the initial screening results. The first step of the simulation model was used to define a cut-off number of four ELISA-positive samples (or 13% of 30 samples) to help differentiate between true- and false-positive flocks. Using that cut-off, the point estimates of flock-level sensitivity and specificity were 99.9% and 99.8%, respectively.

The second step of the simulation showed that the survey was 97.7% sensitive given the survey design and a 1% flock seroprevalence. With that survey, Switzerland would be declared ND seropositive as soon as one flock was found test positive (had more than four individual animal test reactors). The more test positive flocks found, however, the more evidence (or higher likelihood) that Switzerland was truly infected than if only none or just one flock was found test positive. Probability distributions of the number of test-positive flocks expected in a situation of freedom of infection with ND virus compared to a situation where 1% of Swiss flocks would be infected (see Figure 10.4) showed that the survey result of four test-positive flocks was far less likely observed in a situation of freedom than in the nonfree situation. In the simulation approach, only one of 1,000 iterations, representing surveys conducted in a ND-free population, gave a result of four flocks classified as positive. In contrast, this result was observed 158 times out of 1,000 surveys (iterations) conducted in a population with 1% of all flocks infected.

Likelihood ratios (LRs) are sometimes used for the interpretation of animal individual test(s) when results are given on a continuous scale (Fletcher et al. 1996; Smith 1995) to derive a posttest probability of infection for a tested ani-

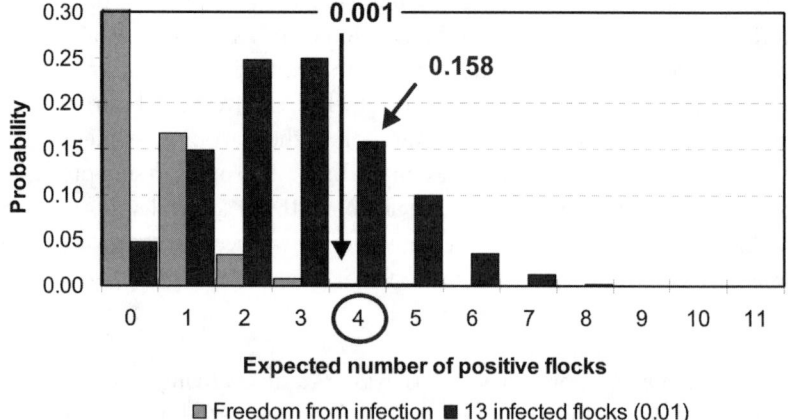

Expected number of positive flocks

☐ Freedom from infection ■ 13 infected flocks (0.01)

FIGURE 10.4   Probability distributions of the number of NCD-positive flocks expected from a serological survey of 260 laying hen flocks in a situation of freedom from Newcastle disease (ND) compared with a situation in which 1% of Swiss flocks would be infected. In this simulation, only one of 1,000 surveys conducted in a ND-free population would give a result of four flocks classified as positive. In contrast, this result would be observed 158 times out of 1,000 surveys conducted in a population with 1% of flocks infected. The actual survey result of four positive flocks provided a likelihood ratio estimate of 0.0063 (1 of 158).

mal. In the context of the ND survey, the LR was defined as the ratio of the probability of observing a specific survey result in the absence of the infection (ND freedom) to the probability of observing the same result in the presence of the infection at a predefined herd prevalence (e.g., 1%).

Other Modeling Approaches

Published practical applications of simulation modeling to assess surveillance activities are currently rare. Paisley et al. (2001) conducted a retrospective analysis of the surveillance programs of infectious bovine rhinotracheitis (IBR) in Norway. IBR is an acute, contagious disease, caused by herpesvirus type I (BHV1), and primarily affecting the upper respiratory tract of cattle. The infection is usually clustered within herds and spreads more slowly between herds following animal movement. Norway had about 25,000 dairy herds and tested about 10% of them between 1996 and 1998, with no positive results. Using stochastic modeling, Paisley et al. (2001) verified that the sampling protocol of 1998 provided a near 99% probability that at least one IBR infected herd would be detected if the disease were present at a herd prevalence of 0.2% (definition of disease freedom according to OIE). Their model was adapted for the use of pooled-serum and bulk-milk testing. The authors considered that 70% of dairy cows would contribute to the bulk-milk sample and that the sensitivity of the ELISA would vary according to the within-herd infection prevalence. Surveys of different size were simulated. After sampling herds from the national population, the number of infected herds in the sample was estimated and the diagnostic status of these infected herds was modeled according to individual herd size and within-herd infection prevalence. No overall herd-level sensitivity was calculated as with Audigé et al. (1999). This approach was similar to the creation of the virtual infected population in the sample size estimator programme of Rüfenacht et al. (2000) presented in a later section.

A similar approach was used to simulate a surveillance program for Johne's disease in Norwegian dairy herds (Paisley et al. 2000). The authors showed that testing using ELISA alone was not a feasible option, thus avoiding the running of a costly and ineffective program. This result highlighted the point made also by other researchers (Audigé et al. 1999; Dargatz et al. 2001; Jordan 1997), that herd freedom certification, in the case of Johne's disease, can not rely on serologic testing alone. Simulation modeling appeared particularly useful in the situation of testing with an imperfect test in low-prevalence herds.

ESTIMATION OF CONFIDENCE IN FREEDOM FROM INFECTION

Simulation modeling has been recently presented as a tool to help substantiate one's confidence in freedom from infection (Audigé et al. 2001). The authors used the surveillance of IBR in Switzerland to illustrate their approach. The simulation model presented above was adapted for the planning and assessment of large surveys involving thousands of herds and animals.

The model allows quantification of the probability (with specific confidence limits) of the absence of infection in a country or a region given specific survey results; that is, the negative predictive value of the survey result (Figure 10.2). Using a Bayesian approach, this probability (defined also as postsurvey probability), is derived from the prior knowledge (i.e., the presurvey probability) of the absence of infection in the country and the likelihood ratio of the survey result as defined with the Newcastle Disease (NCD) example. Fully developed and accepted methods to quantitatively evaluate the presurvey probability of infection freedom are, however, currently lacking.

Simulation modeling was used in the context of two large national Swiss surveys aimed at substantiating freedom from IBR in Switzerland in 1998 and 1999. In the 1998 survey, blood samples were taken from five cattle over 2 years of age in each of 4,672 cattle herds and tested using an ELISA. In 1999, 1% of Swiss herds were selected (i.e., 648 herds), and all cattle more than 2 years in the herd were sampled (Anonymous 1998).

Both surveys had negative test results (i.e., zero positive herds). The likelihood ratio of observing this result under the situation of IBR freedom, compared with the situation of 0.1% infected herds in the population, was 56.7 for the 1998 survey, but only 1.7 for the 1999 survey. Confidence in freedom from IBR was much higher following the 1998 survey than after the 1999 survey when assuming that the prior confidence of freedom (prior probability) was equal for both surveys. This assumption is not fully true: the 1998 survey, when taken as an indicator for the Swiss IBR situation, provided a high pre-1999-probability of IBR freedom. Unfortunately, methods to modify an existing freedom probability over time to account for potential changes (decreases) over time, that is, between two surveys, are also not yet fully developed.

At this stage, it is worth considering the results of the PRRS and NCD surveys presented earlier. All laboratory test results were negative in the PRRS survey. Compared with the modeling outcome (i.e., the survey ROC curve), this result showed that it was extremely unlikely that slaughter pigs in Switzerland were seropositive for PRRS viruses. Given the previous history of absence of PRRS infection in Switzerland, investigators had high confidence, although not quantified in a probabilistic manner, that this country was truly PRRS free.

In the NCD survey, four flocks were classified as positive; that is, they had at least four test-positive birds out of 30. This result provided a LR estimate for freedom for NCD of 0.0063 (1 of 158), which was considered very low. Although very limited prior information was available at the time of the survey, it was concluded that freedom from antibodies against ND viruses of low pathogenicity was highly unlikely.

PREVALENCE ESTIMATION

Prevalence estimation relates to the second required result needed to document the health status of an animal population. Simulation modeling was applied for both the determination of survey sample size and estimation of prevalence. We illustrate these applications in the next sections.

Sample Size Determination

With a simple sampling scheme, the traditional approach is to estimate population prevalence from a randomly selected group of animals. The size of this group can be determined from a prior (even rough) estimate of this prevalence and the absolute or relative precision with which the investigators wish to refine the estimate with a given level of confidence (Canon and Roe 1982; Farver et al. 1985; Lwanga and Lemeshow 1991).

When herd prevalence is estimated, the process of estimation relies on herd-level sampling schemes able to correctly classify infected and noninfected herds. In such cases, the within-herd prevalence of infection is not of direct interest other than to appropriately design a herd-level sampling scheme. The first step of the model of Audigé et al. (2001) presented earlier can be used for that purpose. This is particularly important when animal-level tests with high specificity and sensitivity are not available, such as with Johne's disease. Once the herd-level testing scheme is designed, the number of herds to be sampled can be estimated using a standard approach (i.e., given a prior estimate of herd prevalence, its required precision, and level of confidence).

When trying to estimate animal-level prevalence, however, the fact that infection can cluster within herds brings an additional difficulty. When this clustering effect is large, then the method used for simple sampling without clustering is inadequate because the precision in the estimate drops as the clustering of infection increases. Specific formulae for sample size calculations using cluster sampling for a binomial outcome are available (Thrusfield 1995). However, the calculations require a prior estimation of an intracluster correlation coefficient (Chapter 5), which can be obtained from already-collected cluster sampling data. These calculations may not be very intuitive for most of us. Simulation modeling, however, can provide a more intuitive, objective, and accurate approach.

A program using stochastic simulation was developed to predict optimal sample sizes for one- or two-stage cross-sectional surveys in which clustering of infected animals within herds might be expected (Figure 10.5; Rüfenacht et al. 2000). This model takes into account the total number of herds and the distribution of herd sizes in that population and two parameters: expected overall animal-level prevalence and estimates of within- and between-herd prevalence (which reflects the level of clustering of infected animals within herds). Within

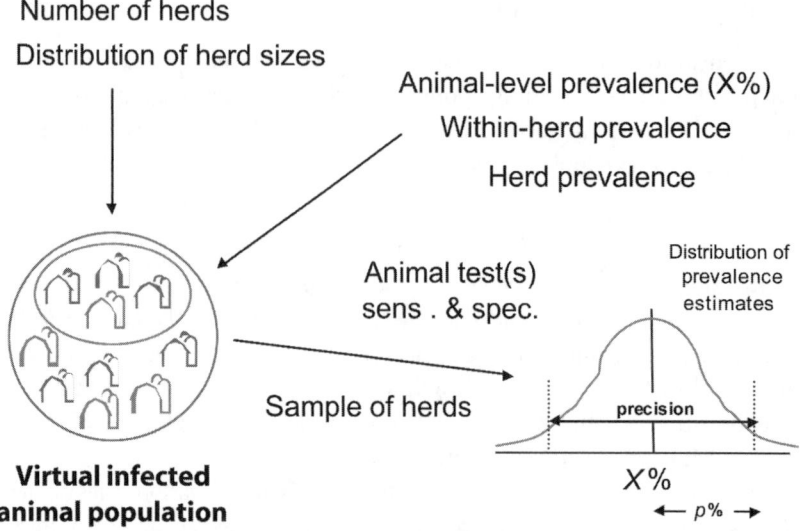

Number of herds
Distribution of herd sizes

Animal-level prevalence (X%)
Within-herd prevalence
Herd prevalence

Animal test(s)
sens . & spec.

Distribution of
prevalence
estimates

Sample of herds

precision

**Virtual infected
animal population**

$X\%$

$\leftarrow p\% \rightarrow$

FIGURE 10.5   Structure of the stochastic model used for sample size calculation in the context of animal-health surveys aimed at estimating animal-level prevalence in the presence of clustering of infection. This program creates a virtual animal population on the basis of the total number of herds and the distribution of herd sizes in that population and two of the following parameters: expected overall animal-level prevalence (first estimate X) and estimates of within- and between-herd prevalence (which reflects the level of clustering of infected animals within herds). Herd sampling and testing, followed by prevalence calculation, is then simulated on that population by successive iterations (virtual surveys). For a range of sample sizes, the distributions of calculated animal-level prevalence are compared. The optimum number of herds to sample in the population is that for which a given percentage of iterations (equivalent to the level of confidence) fall within a given prevalence interval (equivalent to the prevalence estimate $X\%$ and its precision $p\%$).

the model, a virtual population is created on the basis of these parameters. Herd sampling and testing (considering here the animal-level test sensitivity and specificity), followed by calculation of animal-level prevalence, are then simulated on that population by successive iterations. The optimum number of herds to sample in the population is that for which a given percentage of iterations (equivalent to the level of confidence) falls within a given prevalence interval (equivalent to the prevalence estimate and its precision).

A cross-sectional study was conducted in Switzerland to investigate the prevalence of antibodies to bovine viral diarrhea virus (BVDV) in individual animals and of animals persistently infected (PI) with this virus (Rüfenacht et al. 2000). To assess the economic effect of the infection in Switzerland, accurate prevalence estimates based on a survey with appropriately calculated sample size were needed.

Using the simulation program described above, the sampling scheme was designed to account for clustering of persistently infected animals within herds. It was assumed that there would be one to five (most likely four) PI animals in infected herds, with an overall animal prevalence of 3%. The simulation suggested sampling from 110 herds of five to 80 animals (mode of 12 animals) for the estimation of this prevalence with an absolute precision of 1% and a 95% confidence level. The actual survey sampled 121 herds and 3,440 cattle. Simple random sampling calculation would have suggested sampling only 1,120 animals, which would not have given the required precision.

Estimating Prevalence from Survey Results

When conducting surveys, given that the test's sensitivity (Se) and specificity (Sp) are known, a formula can be applied to estimate the true prevalence from the apparent prevalence (AP) given by test results (Marchevsky 1974):

$$\text{True prevalence} = AP + Sp - 1/Se + Sp - 1.$$

This formula was mainly presented for individual-level prevalence, but the same approach can be applied for herd prevalence estimation using simulation modeling to account for parameters' uncertainty (herd-level test sensitivity and specificity) and sampling variation (apparent prevalence). We acknowledge that this formula can produce negative values if AP is very low and the specificity is below 100%. Negative values are usually changed to zero.

In the context of the ND survey presented earlier, as four flocks were classified as positive from 260 flocks sampled, the true prevalence between flocks was estimated. Gohm et al. (1999) reported that this prevalence was around 1.5%, but they did not account for sampling variation. We modeled this prevalence by specifying herd-level sensitivity, herd-level specificity as probability distributions, and apparent prevalence successively as a point estimate (i.e., four of 260, or 1.5%) and as a probability distribution. Resulting flock prevalence distributions provided fairly similar median prevalences at 1.9% and 2.1%, respectively (Figure 10.6). The spread of estimated true prevalence, however, was much larger when sampling variation was taken into account, ranging from 0.2% to 6.3% compared with 1.2%–1.9% otherwise. Sampling variation is an important factor of uncertainty when estimating prevalence of infection, and it relates to the number of units (here flocks) sampled in the survey.

A challenging objective within the framework of surveillance is to estimate the prevalence of infection in a given animal population when the available test(s) detect the infection only in animals in more advanced stages in the incubation period. Stochastic simulation proved useful, for instance, to estimate

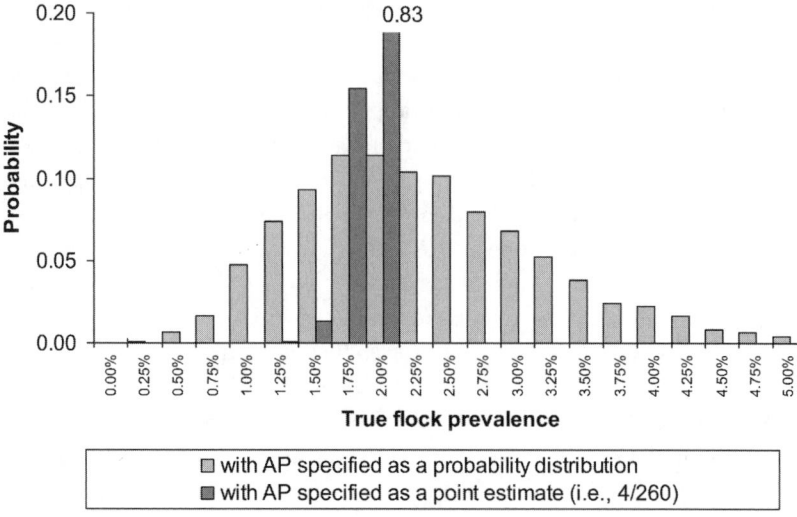

FIGURE 10.6   Stochastic simulation of flock prevalence of infection with lentogenic Newcastle disease viruses in Switzerland in 1996, considering the apparent prevalence as either a point estimate or a probability distribution. Using Marchevsky's formula (1974), the true flock prevalence was estimated by specifying herd-level sensitivity, herd-level specificity, and apparent prevalence as probability distributions. Gohm et al. (1999) reported that the likely flock prevalence of infection was around 1.5%, which is the apparent prevalence (four test-positive flocks out of 260 flocks examined).

the prevalence of sheep scrapie in Great Britain (Webb et al. 2001). The approach implies that a model can be specified to make inferences about the targeted population from the sampled and tested population. In the scrapie example, the development of the infection in sheep and the pattern of slaughtering sheep were modeled. The abattoir survey was designed to estimate a prevalence of detectable infection of 1% with a precision of $\pm$ 0.5% (with 95% confidence); however, all tests were negative. This result was consistent with a prevalence of detectable infection of less than 0.11%. Simulation modeling showed that the same survey result could have been observed if the true infection prevalence at slaughter, including sheep at their early incubation stage, was up to 11%. It was assumed that slaughter was unrelated to scrapie status, but we believe that such a dependency (e.g., in the context of a disease control program) could well be integrated in the modeling process if required.

Such an approach might be particularly useful in the context of other diseases of long incubation period and poor diagnostic ability in the early stage of infection, such as Johne's disease, to identify herds likely to be infected. Animal-health authorities might consider simulation modeling in the framework of eradication or disease-freedom certification programs.

CONCLUSION AND OUTLOOK

Simulation techniques have major strengths for the planning of complex MOSS activities and the interpretation of their results. We supported this view by a series of practical examples, although the approach is currently mostly limited to herd-level sampling schemes and surveys. We envision a broader use of simulation across all MOSS components to optimize their respective strengths and benefits.

The principal advantage of simulation modeling, in comparison to previous approaches, is that it can take into consideration the complexity of disease transmission process and the individual disease-country situations as well as our uncertainty in regard to the current knowledge, or the biologic variability, inherent in the majority of input parameters. Recent advances in computer technology and easy-to-use Monte Carlo–type simulation software packages (such as @Risk, Palisade Corporation, Newfield, NY) have made stochastic simulation readily available.

An important task for groups using this technique will be to communicate simulation results so that they can be understood, accepted, and used. At present, decision makers are likely to rely on confirmatory retesting of animals in the face of (false) positive tests and not on stochastic simulation model outcomes. However, in the ND survey presented earlier, stochastic modeling was in agreement with laboratory retesting in that flocks with up to three test-positive birds were likely to test false-positive. Audigé et al. (1999) speculated that laboratory retesting could be spared following appropriate use of modeling techniques. This will probably depend on the wide acceptance of simulation modeling as a tool for planning MOSS activities and for trusted interpretation of results. Communication issues should therefore be considered carefully.

Compared with more traditional approaches, simulation models can use more of the available information while accounting for uncertainty, which results in a more effective surveillance system. Future development of simulation models should integrate all MOSS components along with economic considerations while using technology to automate the process for end users so that it can be widely applied. Given that investigators understand the value of these methods and have access to reliable epidemiologic data, the planning of animal surveillance systems can be tailored to each targeted animal population and infectious agent and should take into account regional and national differences.

Building on this principle, the Swiss Federal Veterinary Office initiated the use of a risk-based approach for the planning of surveys in its national livestock population (Hadorn 2002; Hauser et al. 2002).

BIBLIOGRAPHY

Anderson R.M., Donnelly C.A., Ferguson N.M., Woolhouse M.E., Watt C.J., Udy H.J., MaWhinney S., Dunstan S.P., Southwood T.R., Wilesmith J.W., Ryan J.B., Hoinville L.J., Hillerton J.E., Austin A.R., Wells G.A. 1996. Transmission dynamics and epidemiology of BSE in British cattle. Nature 382:779–788.

Anonymous. 1998. Council directive of 24 June 1998 amending Annexes A, D (Chapter I) and F to Directive 64/432/EEC on health problems affecting intra-Community trade in bovine animals and swine, 98/46/EC, OJ No. L 198, 15.07.98, p 22.

Audigé L., Beckett, S. 1999. A quantitative assessment of the validity of animal-health surveys using stochastic modelling. Prev Vet Med 38:259–276.

Audigé L., Wagner B., Salman M. 1999. A quantitative assessment of the validity of herd-level testing schemes for Johnes' disease in the USA. Is serological testing sufficient? Proceedings of the Seventy-Ninth meeting of the Conference of Research Workers in Animal Diseases, November 1999. Chicago. Iowa State University Press, Ames, IA, Abstract 58.

Audigé L., Doherr M.G., Hauser R., Salman M.D. 2001. Stochastic modelling as a tool for planning animal health surveys and interpreting screening test results. Prev Vet Med 49:1–17

Cameron A.R. 2002. Survey toolbox; http://www.ausvet.com.au/.

Cameron A.R., Baldock F.C. 1998a. A new probability formula for surveys to substantiate freedom from disease. Prev Vet Med 34:1–17.

Cameron A.R., Baldock F.C. 1998b. Two-stage sampling in surveys to substantiate freedom from disease. Prev Vet Med 34:19–30.

Cannon R.M. 2001. Sense and sensitivity—Designing surveys based on an imperfect test. Prev Vet Med 49:141–163.

Cannon R.M., Roe R.T. 1982. Livestock disease surveys: A field manual for veterinarians. Australian Government Publishing Service, Canberra.

Canon N., Audigé L., Denac H., Hofmann M., Griot C. 1998. Evidence of freedom from porcine reproductive and respiratory syndrome (PRRS) virus infection in Switzerland. Vet Rec 142:142–143

Carpenter T.E., McBride M.D., Hird D.W. 1998. Risk analysis of quarantine station performance: A case study of the importation of equine infectious anemia virus-infected horses into California. J Vet Diag Invest 10:11–16.

Carpenter T.E., Gardner I.A. 1996. Simulation modeling to determine herd-level predictive values and sensitivity based on individual-animal test sensitivity and specificity and sample size. Prev Vet Med 27:57–66.

Dargatz D.A., Byrum B.A., Barber L.K., Sweeney R.W., Whitlock R.H., Shulaw W.P., Jacobson R.H., Stabel J.R. 2001. Evaluation of a commercial ELISA for diagnosis of paratuberculosis in cattle. J Am Vet Med Assoc 218:1163–1166.

Doherr M.G., Audigé L. 2001. Monitoring and surveillance for rare health-related events—A review from the veterinary perspective, in population biology of emerging and re-emerging pathogens. Philos Trans R Soc B 356:1097–1106.

Donald A.W. 1993. Prevalence estimation using diagnostic tests when there are multiple, correlated disease states in the same animal or farm. Prev Vet Med 15:125–145.

Donald A.W., Gardner I.A., Wiggins A.D. 1994. Cut-off points for aggregate herd testing in the presence of disease clustering and correlation of test errors. Prev Vet Med 19:167–187.

Dufour B. and Audigé L. 1997. A proposed classification of veterinary epidemiosurveillance networks. Rev Sci Technique 16:746–758

Farver T.B., Thomas C., Edson R. 1985. An application of sampling theory in animal disease prevalence survey design. Prev Vet Med 3:463–473.

Fletcher R.H., Fletcher S.W., Wagner E.H. 1996. Clinical epidemiology: The essentials. Williams & Wilkins, Baltimore, MD.

Gohm D., Thür B., Audigé L., Hofmann M. 1999. Serological testing and simulation modeling: A survey of Newcastle disease in Swiss laying hen flocks. Prev Vet Med 38:277–288.

Greiner M., Pfeiffer D., Smith R.D. 2000. Principles and practical application of the receiver-operating characteristic analysis for diagnostic tests. Prev Vet Med 45:23–41.

Hadorn D. 2002. Risk-based design of repeated surveys for the documentation of freedom from disease in national livestock populations in Switzerland. University of Bern, Bern, Switzerland, Dissertation 2002.

Hauser R., Hadorn D., Rüfenacht J., Stärk K.D.C. 2002. Examens par sondages permettant d'établir que la Suisse est indemne de certaines epizooties. Epidémiol Santé Anim, in press.

Hurd H.S., Kaneene J.B. 1993. The application of simulation models and systems analysis in epidemiology: A review. Prev Vet Med 15:81–99.

Jordan D. 1997. Aggregate testing for the evaluation of Johne's disease herd status. Aust Vet J 73:16–19.

Jordan D., McEwen S.A. 1998. Herd-level test performance based on uncertain estimates of individual test performance, individual true prevalence and herd true prevalence. Prev Vet Med 36:187–209.

Keeling M.J., Woolhouse M.E.J., Shaw D.J., Matthews L., Chase-Topping M., Haydon D.T., Cornell S.J., Kappey J., Wilesmith J., Grenfell B.T. 2001. Dynamics of the 2001 UK foot and mouth rpidemic: Stochastic dispersal in a heterogeneous landscape. Science 294:813–817.

Loh W.-L. 1996. On Latin Hypercube sampling. Ann Stat 24:2058–2080.

Lwanga S.K., Lemeshow S. 1991. Sample size determination in health studies—A practical manual. World Health Organization, Geneva.

Marchevsky N. 1974. Errors in prevalence estimates in population studies: A practical method for calculating real prevalence. Zoonosis 16:98–109.

Martin S.W., Meek A.H., Willeberg P. 1987. Veterinary epidemiology—Principles and methods. Ames, Iowa, USA, Iowa State University Press, 343 pages.

Martin S.W., Shoukri M., Thorburn M.A. 1992. Evaluating the health status of herds based on tests applied to individuals. Prev Vet Med 14:33–43.

Meredith M. 1995. Review of the worldwide PRRS literature. Pig Disease Information Centre, University of Cambridge, Boehringer Ingelheim Vetmedica GmbH. University of Cambridge, Cambridge, United Kingdom.

Ministry of Agriculture and Fisheries. 2002. Animal and Animal Product Risk Analyses, MAF Biosecurity, New Zealand Ministry of Agriculture and Fisheries; http://www.maf.govt.nz/biosecurity/pests-diseases/animals/risk/index.htm.

Moore D.R.J. 1996. Using Monte Carlo Analysis to quantify uncertainty in ecological risk assessment: Are we eliding the lily or bronzing the dandelilon? Human Ecol Risk Assess 2:628–633.

Morris R.S., Wilesmith J.W., Stern M.W., Sanson R.L., Stevenson M.A. 2001. Predictive spatial modelling of alternative control strategies for the foot-and-mouth disease epidemic in Great Britain, 2001. Vet Rec 149:137–144.

Paisley L.G., Tharaldsen J., Jarp J. 2000. A simulated surveillance program for bovine paratuberculosis in dairy herds in Norway. Prev Vet Med 44:141–151.

Paisley L.G., Tharaldsen J., Jarp J. 2001. A retrospective analysis of the infectious bovine rhinotracheitis (bovine herpes virus-1) surveillance program in Norway using Monte Carlo simulation models. Prev Vet Med 50:109–125.

Rüfenacht J., Schaller P., Audigé L., Strasser, M., Peterhans E. 2000. Prevalence of cattle infected with bovine viral diarrhoea virus in Switzerland. Vet Rec 147:413–417.

Rugen P., Callahan B. 1996. An overview of Monte Carlo, a fifty year perspective. Human Ecol Risk Assess 2:671–680.

Smith R.D. 1995. Veterinary clinical epidemiology—A problem-oriented approach, 2nd ed. CRC Press, London.

Thrusfield M. 1995. Veterinary Epidemiology, 2nd ed. Blackwell Science.

Toma B., Dufour B., Sanaa M., Bénet J.J., Ellis P., Moutou F., Louzã A. 2000. épidémiologie appliquée à la lutte collective contre les maladies animales transmissibles majeures, 2nd ed. AEEMA, France.

Vose D. 1996. Quantitative risk analysis—A guide to Monte Carlo simulation modelling. Wiley, Chichester.

Vose D. 1997. Risk analysis in relation to the importation and exportation of animal products. Rev Sci Technique 16:17–29.

Wagner B., Salman M. 2000. Aggregate testing in veterinary medicine: Overview of previous work and options. Proceedings of the Ninth International Symposium on Veterinary Epidmiology and Economics. August 2000. Breckenridge, CO; CDROM paper 618

Webb C.R., Wilesmith J.W., Simmons M.M., Hoinville L.J. 2001. A stochastic model to estimate the prevalence of scrapie in Great Britain using the results of an abattoir-based survey. Prev Vet Med 51:269–287.

World Trade Organization. 1995. Agreement on the Application of Sanitary and Phytosanitary Measures, World Trade Organization; http://www.wto.org.

Zepeda C., Salman M., Ruppanner R. 2001. International trade, animal health and veterinary epidemiology: Challenges and opportunities. Prev Vet Med 48:261–271.

Quality Assessment of Animal Disease Surveillance and Survey Systems

K.D.C. Stärk

INTRODUCTION

Surveillance programs and surveys are implemented for specific purposes. The data generated are to be used to document the health status of a livestock population and to trigger action. Often the objective is also, in accordance with the Agreement on the Application of Sanitary and Phytosanitary Measures (SPS) of the World Trade Organization, to facilitate trade. Thus, it is essential that the data delivered by animal surveillance systems and surveys are of sufficient quality to satisfy the demands of trading partners or other data users.

Quality assurance and evaluation methods do therefore need to be applied to every animal monitoring and surveillance system (MOSS). The question of quality needs to be addressed at the point of designing a MOSS, but also later by users of the system output. This chapter will suggest a set of methods and approaches for the evaluation of the quality of surveillance and survey systems.

Swiss Federal Veterinary Office
CH-3003 Bern
Switzerland

OBJECTIVES OF QUALITY ASSESSMENTS

The objectives of the assessment should be clearly defined before the task is commenced. A MOSS can be assessed in terms of its quality independently, or several systems can be compared in terms of their relative quality (Box 11.1).

Under the SPS, the question of equivalence is a relevant issue, as importing countries have the right to define the appropriate level of sanitary protection and to request that the exporting country applies equivalent sanitary measures. How the equivalent level of protection is reached, however, is likely to differ among countries. The *Codex Alimentarius Commission* has been dealing with this issue and recommends that to reach a judgment, a "transparent analytical process that is objective and consistent" should be used (Anonymous 2001).

This requirement can be formulated more generally. No matter for what purpose the assessment is conducted, a systematic, objective, and transparent approach needs to be used.

APPROACHES TO QUALITY ASSESSMENTS

The first step of the assessment is a detailed description of the system. The description needs to include the purpose and operation of the system (e.g., the

Box 11.1

Possible motivations for quality assessments of monitoring and surveillance systems (MOSSs):

1 Designing of a new MOSS (by MOSS "owner")
2 Improvement of an existing MOSS (by MOSS "owner")
   • Improving quality
   • IImproving cost-effectiveness
3 Decision on acceptance of data produced by a MOSS (by MOSS "user")
4 Determination of equivalence between MOSS in the context of international trade

Possible questions asked at the start of a quality assessment of a MOSS:

1 Is the MOSS good enough to achieve its purpose?
2 Are the data and results produced by a MOSS of sufficient quality?
3 How could a MOSS be improved?
4 Is MOSS A preferable to MOSS B?
5 Are MOSS A and B equivalent?

objectives, the event under surveillance [case definition], the legal basis, the authorities involved and their responsibilities, and the components of the system) and the resources. Once the description is available, the assessment can proceed. Basically, graphical, textual, and numeric approaches are available for the assessment of a MOSS. As MOSSs may be complex, it may be necessary to use a combination of methods (Figure 11.1).

Detailed protocols for the evaluation of epidemiological surveillance systems have been developed by the World Health Organization (WHO) and by the Centers for Disease Control and Prevention (CDC; CDC 2001; Thacker et al. 1988). The person or team applying this protocol needs to have considerable expertise and competence in the field of MOSS. The key activity in this approach is to gather credible evidence regarding the performance of the system. This also starts with the description of the system. A set of attributes were defined to structure the evaluation of the system capacity (Box 11.2). Evidence is collected from persons or documents or through observations. The evidence is then organized, analyzed, and interpreted. Eventually, this leads to a final judgment. The output of this type of evaluation will be a report and a set of recommendations.

The most challenging process during the evaluation is the analysis of the evidence. It is important to organize the information such that patterns and important findings can be identified. Fault trees are one graphical tool used in the processing industry to identify series of events that will lead to an undesired event (fault). They are useful for an in-depth description of a complex system with the objective of identifying things that can go wrong. This method has a top-down structure with branches being connected with so-called "and" and "or" gates. At an "and" gate, both conditions leading to the gate have to be fulfilled for the event to happen. At an "or" gate, either of the conditions or both

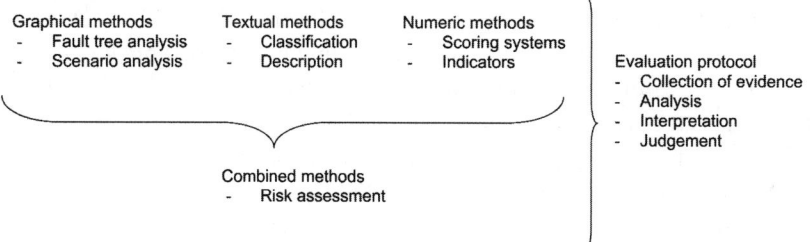

FIGURE 11.1 Approaches to the evaluation of quality of a monitoring and surveillance system.

Box 11.2

Scoring system to assess the quality of monitoring and surveillance systems (MOSSs) for exotic diseases (simplified from Dufour 1999):

		Maximum Score
1	Aims	15
2	Sampling	20
3	Coordination and awareness	15
4	Environmental factors	4
5	Screening and diagnosis	20
6	Data collection and transfer	10
7	Data processing and analysis	10
8	Information dissemination	6
	TOTAL	100

may be true. Fault trees can be used to investigate events leading to unsatisfactory quality of MOSS. See Figure 11.2 for suggested elements of a fault tree leading to inadequate quality of MOSS. Of particular interest are "and" gates.

The advantage of the fault tree is that it supports a systematic and complete analysis of the system. In addition, it helps us to understand interactions between events and their influence on quality. Fault trees are particularly useful to identify weaknesses in a system. They have also been criticized because of this, as they may overemphasize the negative aspects of a system. Decision makers who are not familiar with fault trees may then overestimate the probability that the undesirable top event, in our case, unsatisfactory quality of a system, will occur.

A second graphical approach is scenario analysis. A scenario is a chronology of events that can occur when starting with a given event; for example, the occurrence of a case to be registered in a MOSS. Given the design of a MOSS, the subsequent events (e.g., detection of case, sampling, confirmation of case, and reporting of case) can be determined and integrated. This method is suitable for the structured description of a complex MOSS and can also be used quantitatively if the necessary data are available (Hueston and Yoe 2000).

Another possible method is the characterization of MOSS through its elements (objectives, target population[s], designing issues related to sampling scheme and organization, diagnostic methods, data management, analysis, feedback, and dissemination of results). These can be used for assessing the MOSS according to classification rules. Such a classification may be useful for the direct comparison of surveillance systems, such as in the context of assess-

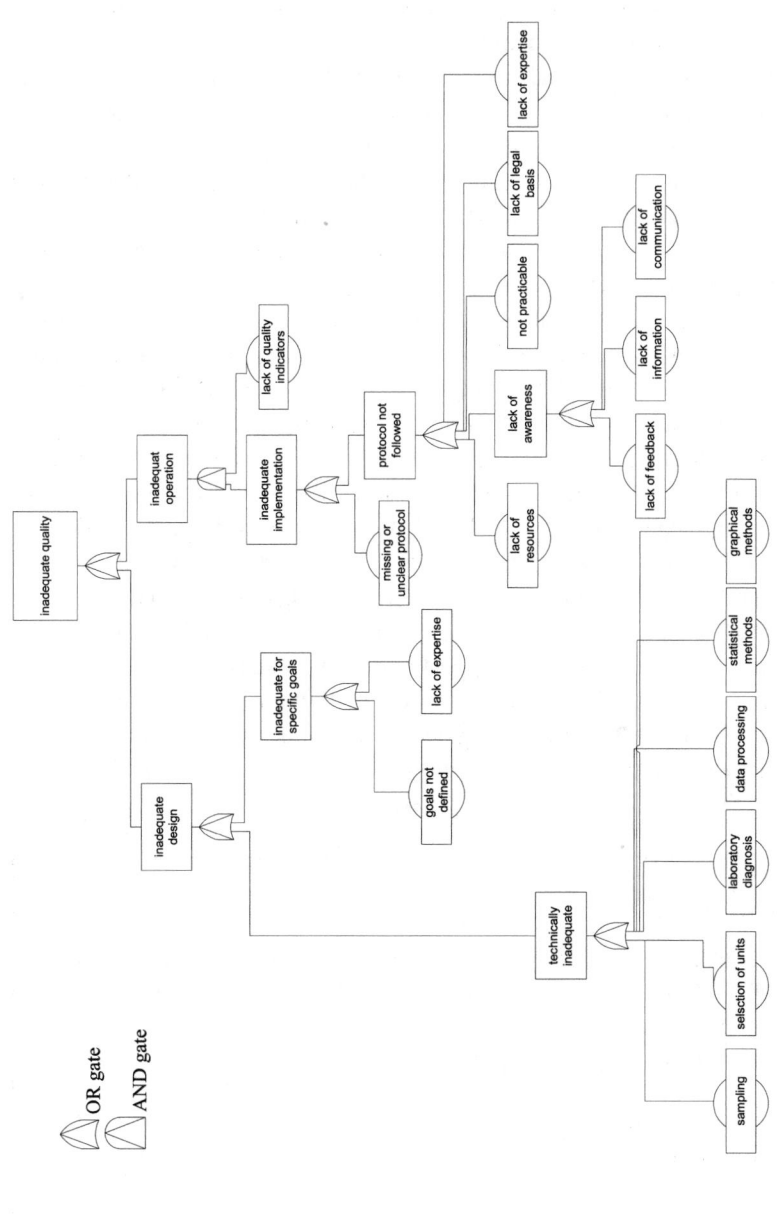

OR gate

AND gate

FIGURE 11.2   Fault tree example for events leading to inadequate quality of a monitoring and surveillance system.

173

ing the degree of equivalence of systems applied in different countries. However, the result will be limited in that equivalence in quality can still exist although the systems may not be composed of exactly the same elements. However, the equivalence of design and structure is not necessarily sufficient to determine equivalence in quality.

Fault trees, scenario analyses, and classification of MOSS may be suitable for the descriptive assessment of a system and for simple comparisons of several MOSSs. However, in some instances, quantitative information may be required. For this purpose, scoring systems have been suggested that express results as quality scores (Dufour 1999). With this method, critical control points of MOSS are marked (Box 11.3). A maximum score is assigned for each control point, thus weighting their relative importance, and with a total adding up to 100 points. When evaluating a MOSS, a detailed manual is used to determine the actual score for each element. This procedure allows the identification of the weaknesses of a MOSS. The end score of several MOSS can be directly compared, with the system with the higher score being the better one.

Quantitative information can also be derived by using quality or performance indicators. Performance indicators have been used as quality assurance tools integrated in the design of MOSS; for example, in the global rinderpest eradication program (Anonymous 2000). Often, performance indicators are simple ratios or proportions that can be measured against a defined target. The indicators can also be used for comparison between several MOSSs provided that they are general enough to apply to different designs.

As a MOSS often is a complex structure with numerous components and, therefore, many factors influencing quality, a combination of the methods and approaches described above may have to be used. The concept of risk assess-

Box 11.3

Attributes to consider when evaluating the capacity of a monitoring and surveillance system:

1 Sensitivity
2 Specificity
3 Predictive values
4 Representativeness
5 Timeliness
6 Simplicity
7 Flexibility
8 Acceptability
9 Consistency

ment may be useful in this context, as it is essentially a framework for organizing information in a standardized way to reach a synthesis of the evidence. If the quality of a MOSS is defined as sufficient if the risk of certain events is smaller than a target value, the risk assessment approach can easily be translated to this problem. As in other contexts, the risk assessment would involve the identification of hazards or hazardous events, the description of scenario pathways leading to an undesired event, the collection of evidence, and finally, a qualitative or quantitative assessment of the probability of this event and its consequences including the related uncertainty. This approach is now routinely used by importing countries to assess the risk of introduction of infectious agents through the importation of food, animals, or plants.

RELEVANCE OF QUALITY FOR MOSS "OWNERS"

Quality assurance should be an integral part of the design of a MOSS to assure that it is capable of serving its purpose. Quality assurance systems have been developed in many processing and production industries. Such programs are now widely used. Some general principles are equally applicable to quality assurance of MOSS. Among these principles are the need for documentation and the need for monitoring.

Documentation is a *sine qua non* requirement for a later evaluation of the quality of a MOSS. All protocols on methods and procedures have to be written down in detail. This includes all steps of sampling, sample processing, data recording, laboratory analyses, and statistical analysis. Particularly in the case of multicenter data collection, a written manual with detailed instructions for all participating parties is desirable.

The performance of MOSS can also be monitored through routine procedures set down in the design document. Performance indicators can be defined for certain aspects of a system. For example, the number of disease reports from districts received within a target time period could be such an indicator. These indicators can then be calculated regularly and be monitored for increasing or decreasing trends.

If quality assurance mechanisms are inherent parts of MOSS, their evaluation by MOSS "users" is facilitated considerably. A fully documented system can also be audited easily. This is comparable with a repeated evaluation of the quality of the system.

CONCLUSIONS

The assessment of the quality of MOSS is a routine task conducted by both the MOSS "owners" as well as the "users." Various approaches are available, the suitability of which depends on the objective of the evaluation. An essential basic requirement is, however, to use an objective, transparent, and systematic approach. The evidence collected and the analyses used to reach conclusions need to be such that the results are acceptable to the management of the MOSS as well as to the assessor. Repeated discussions and negotiations may be necessary to reach consensus, particularly if the judgment affects activities between trading partners. Well-documented MOSSs with specified objectives and integrated quality assurance mechanisms are likely to be easier to evaluate.

SUGGESTED FURTHER READINGS

Centers for Disease Control and Prevention. 1999. Framework for program evaluation in public health. Morbid Mort Wkly Rep 48:PP-11.
World Health Organization. 1997. Protocol for the evaluation of epidemiological surveillance systems. Geneva, WHO/EMC/DIS/97.2.

BIBLIOGRAPHY

Anonymous. 2000. Guidelines for the use of performance indicators in rinderpest surveillance programmes. International Atomic Energy Agency, Vienna, IAEA-TECDOC-1161.
Anonymous. 2001. Proposed draft guidelines on the judgment of equivalence of sanitary measures associated with food inspection and certification systems. Codex Alimentarius Commission, Rome, ALINORM 01/30A, Appendix III.
Centers for Disease Control and Prevention. 2001. Updated guidelines for evaluating public health systems. Morb Mort Wkly Rep 50:PP-13.
Dufour, B. 1999. Technical and economic evaluation method for use in improving infectious animal disease surveillance networks. Vet Rese 30:27–37.
Hueston, W.D., Yoe, C.E. 2000. Estimating the overall power of complex surveillance systems. Proceedings of Ninth International Symposium of Veterinary Epidemiology and Economics, August 5–11, 2000. Breckinridge, CO, pp 758–760.
Thacker S.B., Parrish R.G., Trowbridge F.L. 1988. A method for evaluating systems of epidemiological surveillance. World Health Stat Q 41:11–18.

Dissemination of Surveillance Findings

N.E. Wineland and D.A. Dargatz

INTRODUCTION

In general, a monitoring or surveillance system (MOSS) is of little value if the information gathered is not distributed to decision makers and is not oriented toward action. Dissemination of information is best accomplished through careful consideration of the intended audience and the most efficient and effective means of reaching the intended audience. The information must be packaged in a form that can be readily assimilated and used. If it is expected or hoped that the surveillance findings will lead to action, the information must be targeted to those who will take the action as well as to those who will want the action taken.

A variety of approaches may be taken to disseminate information, and these will be explored in this chapter. In the United States, the National Animal Health Monitoring System (NAHMS) was established to collect, analyze, and report on

Centers for Epidemiology and Animal Health
Natural Resources Research Center, Bldg B
2150 Centre Avenue, Mail Stop 2W6
Fort Collins, CO 80526–8117

animal health and has evolved to include interactions of animal health, animal production, animal welfare, product wholesomeness, and the environment (http://www.aphis.usda.gov/vs/ceah/cahm/). The reporting approaches covered in this chapter will be drawn from the experiences of the NAHMS program, with emphasis on the strengths and limitations of each option.

For purposes of discussion reports will be divided into two categories. Internal reports are those that are geared to individuals intimately involved in the surveillance effort. This audience has significant knowledge of the design of the surveillance system and the underlying processes being monitored such that detailed background information and explanations are unnecessary in reports of findings. The information may need limited interpretation to be actionable for this internal audience, and the dissemination process can be expedited when explanatory interpretive narratives are not required. External reports are those destined for an audience not familiar with the surveillance approach or the processes being monitored and therefore include more details on the background, data collection methods, analysis, and interpretation of the findings. Although there is much overlap between these categories, it is useful to consider dissemination efforts in light of audience familiarity with the surveillance system.

INTERNAL REPORTS

Internal reports are limited in their distribution and are most appropriately used when the findings of surveillance are intended for use with an audience that is intimately familiar with the surveillance system. Such reports are appropriate when the data and content of the reports are of a confidential nature.

Internal reports can take a variety of forms, ranging from internal memos to documents in a format more similar to external reports.

EXTERNAL REPORTS

Like internal reports, external reports can take on many forms. The difference is that the intended audience includes those not directly involved with the surveillance effort. In general, these reports need to include more explanation of the design of the surveillance system, monitoring program, or survey, as the audience may have less familiarity with the approach. In developing these reports, it may be that each targeted audience will need to have a slightly different report to be sure that the intended message is clear to the recipient and that the information needed for action is present in a useable form.

Descriptive reports are generally used to give tabular summaries of the gathered information for the population under a MOSS (Figure 12.1). Depending on the needs of the audience, descriptive reports can also include graphic representations of the findings. In the NAHMS system, the audience for the descriptive reports includes academicians, epidemiologists, and others with a high level of knowledge about the included topics and surveillance. These reports tend to serve as a reference document for all the findings of a particular surveillance effort. A disadvantage of this type of report is that although attempts are made to help the reader interpret some of the information, the interpretation of the bulk of the surveillance information is left to the reader. There is limited opportunity in this format to include comments on the limitations of the surveillance system or data. Even if such comments are included, it is easy for a reader to focus on the tabular presentation without appreciating the limitations of what is being presented. When limited interpretation will be done by those conducting the surveillance, extra effort is required to be sure that table headings and figure legends are clear and to make the technical experts available for consultation should there be questions.

Interpretive reports, as the name would imply, include a substantial amount of interpretation of the data. Under the NAHMS scheme, we have used interpretive reports to include all information relevant to a particular topic along with an in-depth narrative of the system design, data analysis, results, and interpretation. This type of report has an advantage over descriptive reports in that all of the pertinent related information is in one complete report. In the NAHMS setting in which each project is often conducted in a multistage design, these reports may take longer to create if all of the relevant data are gathered in multiple stages.

Another kind of external report used in the NAHMS system is the trends report (Figure 12.2). This type of report is used to describe changes occurring over time. To generate this type of report, the same or very similar data must be gathered from the same or similar respondents over time. Otherwise, it is difficult to make comparisons over time if there are changes in either the data collection instrument or the respondent profile.

Information sheets are another type of external report (Figure 12.3). In the case of NAHMS, these are used when the intended audience may not have a high level of knowledge on the particular topics. Information sheets are meant to be a succinct discussion of the project findings with regard to a very specific topic area. They include much more in the way of explanatory details and less emphasis on the system design and far fewer tabular representations of information than are found in descriptive reports.

In addition, external reports may also include refereed journal articles, abstracts or posters given at professional or industry meetings, lay press news

Costs of treating disease conditions

Es ti mates of costs to treat one sick ani mal in the table be low in cluded costs of medi cines and re lated items, such as sy ringes, but did not in clude vet eri nary, la bor, or other, simi lar charges. Retreatment costs were also in cluded.

Acute interstitial pneumo nia, res pi ra tory dis eases, and cen tral nerv ous sys tem problems had the high est costs to treat one sick ani mal. Treat ment costs for both respiratory categories were higher for larger feed lots than small feed lots ($16.26 com pared to $11.09 for res pi ra tory dis ease and $16.49 compared to $11.87 for acute interstitial pneumonia).

a. Operation average medicine costs (in dollars) to treat one sick animal for the following medical conditions by feedlot capacity:

Medical Condition	Operation Average Cost (In Dollars)					
	Feedlot Capacity (Number Head)				All Feedlots	
	1,000 - 7,999		8,000 or More			
	Cost	Standard Error	Cost	Standard Error	Cost	Standard Error
Respiratory disease such as shipping fever	$11.09	($0.62)	$16.26	($0.77)	$12.59	($0.49)
Acute interstitial pneumonia	$11.87	($0.58)	$16.49	($0.86)	$13.33	($0.48)
Digestive problems (excluding non-eaters)	$6.14	($0.83)	$6.27	($0.36)	$6.19	($0.56)
Bullers	$0.86	($0.18)	$1.55	($0.23)	$1.10	($0.14)
Lameness	$7.03	($0.71)	$9.24	($0.55)	$7.68	($0.53)
Central nervous system problems	$11.61	($1.02)	$11.29	($0.71)	$11.50	($0.72)

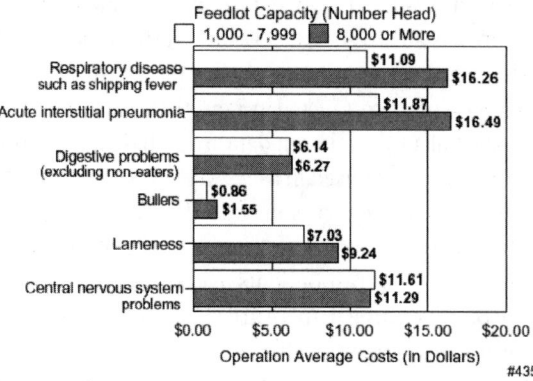

Operation Average Medicine Costs to Treat One Sick Animal for the Following Medical Conditions by Feedlot Capacity

#4358

FIGURE 12.1   Example page from a descriptive report of the United States National Animal Health Information System.

items, books and book chapters, and Web-based publications. Some of these methods of information release can be more time consuming than the production of an internal or external report. Journal articles must undergo a peer review process, and often, the length of time it takes for an article to be accepted for publication can be prolonged. However, it may be the best way to

The best way to categorize cause of death in a feedlot animal is via a postmortem examination (autopsy/necropsy). Postmortems can be effectively performed by veterinarians or trained feedlot personnel. Failure to do postmortems will likely result in some misclassification of animal deaths and may lead to the inability to identify trends in cattle health such as treatment failure, misdiagnosis of live animals, or seasonal peaks in the incidence of diseases such as acute interstitial pneumonia.

There was a substantial increase in the percentage of dead cattle that had a postmortem examination from 1994 (45.9 percent) to 1999 (53.9 percent). This increase was primarily from postmortems by non-veterinarians.

b. Percent of dead cattle where a postmortem examination was done during the year by:				
	1994 COFE		Feedlot '99	
Examiner	Percent	Standard Error	Percent	Standard Error
A veterinarian	15.5	(1.5)	13.2	(0.7)
A nonveterinarian	30.4	(2.4)	40.7	(2.1)
No postmortem performed	54.1	(2.5)	46.1	(2.3)
Total	100.0		100.0	

Percent of Dead Cattle Where a Postmortem Examination Was Done by Examiner, 1994 and 1999

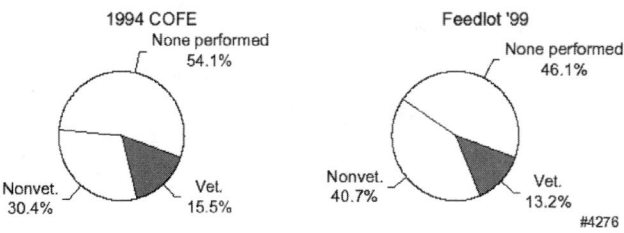

FIGURE 12.2   Example page from a trends report of the United States National Animal Health Monitoring System.

reach a particular audience, and it allows all of the methods and analysis approaches to be fully described. Advantages of the journal articles include the critical review of the methods and interpretation of the results that come with the peer review process and the archival of the findings for the scientific community. Because many of the peer-reviewed articles are included by the abstracting services, the articles become searchable and accessible to anyone in the world. Books and book chapters may reach key audiences as well and are often used in conjunction with other methods. Abstracts and posters are faster in disseminating information than are journal articles and books, but they may reach a smaller audience. Lay press news items and Web-based publications are likely the fastest means for disseminating findings and rely on the tremendous multiplier effect that these publications can have. Because the media can have a substantial readership, providing the information to one of these outlets can

INFO SHEET
APHIS

United States Department of Agriculture
Animal and Plant Health Inspection Service
October 2001

Veterinary Services

Salmonella in United States Feedlots

Salmonella is a significant cause of foodborne illness in the U.S., resulting in an estimated 1.3 million human cases, 15,600 hospitalizations, and 550 deaths each year[1].

The beef industry has implemented many intervention strategies in harvest facilities to reduce the likelihood of carcass contamination with *Salmonella* and other potential foodborne pathogens.

In addition to these post-harvest strategies, there continues to be interest in pre-harvest strategies for reducing the pathogen loads in the gastrointestinal tracts of animals or on the hides of animals presented for harvest. To understand the potential for pre-harvest intervention, it is important to understand the distribution of these pathogens in the feedlot setting.

In 1999, the USDA's National Animal Health Monitoring System (NAHMS) conducted Feedlot '99, a study of feedlots with 1,000-head-or-more capacity within the 12 leading cattle feeding states (Figure 1). These operations represented 84.9 percent of the U.S. feedlots in 1999 and contained 96.1 percent of the U.S. cattle inventory on feedlots with 1,000-head-or-more capacity on January 1, 2000.

As part of this study, 73 feedlots were recruited to collect fecal samples from pen floors throughout a one-year period (October 1999 through September 2000). In each feedlot, 25 fecal samples were collected from the floors of three pens. The pens were selected to represent cattle that had been on feed the shortest time, the longest time, and a randomly selected pen (75 total samples). Sampling occurred in each feedlot twice over the course of the year.

Overall, 6.3 percent of fecal samples were positive for *Salmonella*. There was little difference in the percentage of samples positive for *Salmonella* by type of pen (Table 1).

The percentage of culture-positive samples collected within a pen ranged from 0 to 100. However, the median percentage of samples positive from all pens was 0. For pens that had at least one positive sample, the median percentage of samples positive was 14.

Figure 1.
Twelve Leading Cattle Feeding States

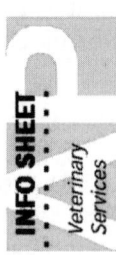

The largest percentage of samples was positive (11.4 percent) in the fourth sampling period, July through September (Figure 1).

Table 1. Percent Samples Positive for *Salmonella*, by Pen Type

Pen type	Samples collected	Samples positive	Percent samples positive
Short-fed	3,482	212	6.1
Random	3,400	217	6.4
Long-fed	3,485	224	6.4
Unknown	50	1	2.0
Total	10,417	654	6.3

Figure 2.
Percent Samples Positive For *Salmonella*, by Season

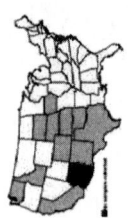

The percentage of samples positive for *Salmonella* differed by the geographic region[2] of the feedlot. Samples from Southern operations were more likely to test positive (7.7 percent) than samples from Northern operations (4.8 percent).

Overall, 22.3 percent (94/422) of pens had one or more positive samples. The 94 positive pens were located in 50.7 percent (37/73) of feedlots where samples were collected.

In this study, the most common serotypes of *Salmonella* recovered from samples collected from feedlot pen floors were dissimilar from those most commonly associated with human illness or cattle diagnostic specimens, with the exception of *S. newport* (Table 2).

Table 2. Five Most Common Serotypes of *Salmonella*, from Various Sources

Serotypes from humans (1996)[a]	Serotypes from cattle (1999/2000)[a]	Serotypes from cattle feedlots (1999/2000)
Typhimurium	Typhimurium	Anatum
Enteritidis	Anatum	Montevideo
Newport	Dublin	Reading
Heidelberg	Montevideo	Newport
Muenchen	Newport	Kentucky

[a] Source: CDC data
[b] Source: USDA-APHIS-VS National Veterinary Service Laboratories

Future analyses of these data will focus on animal and nutritional factors associated with samples from pens testing positive and the antimicrobial susceptibility patterns of *Salmonella* isolates.

For more information contact:
Centers for Epidemiology and Animal Health
USDA-APHIS, attn. NAHMS
555 South Howes
Fort Collins, CO 80521, (970) 490-8000
NAHMSweb@aphis.usda.gov
www.aphis.usda.gov/vs/ceah/cahm

#N346.1001

[1] Mead et al., Food-related Illness and Death in the United States. Emerg. Inf. Dis. 5:607–625

[2] **Northern Region:** Idaho, Iowa, Kansas, Nebraska, South Dakota, Washington
Southern Region: California, Colorado, New Mexico, Oklahoma, Texas

FIGURE 12.3   Example of an info sheet that is used by the United States Animal Health Information System.

result in extremely wide distribution of the information. Both require information to be packaged in a ready-to-use format. Good relationships with editors of industry publications and recognition by major search engines are paramount to maximizing the effectiveness of this route of dissemination. A downside to this route is that it may preclude the possibility of publication in a refereed journal. In addition, there are often limitations to the amount of background on the methods that can be included in the news releases.

Release of information on a Web site can be a very rapid way to reach a broad audience that has access to the Internet. This approach can be extremely cost efficient as long as the intended audience is likely to have access to the World Wide Web, and there are ways to make the intended audience aware of the availability of the new information.

DISSEMINATION OF FINDINGS

During the planning stages for a project or surveillance system, it is useful to consider each intended audience separately, paying particular attention to who will take action based on the information generated. Each audience may need a separate report targeted to the issues and expertise of the group. In our experience with the NAHMS, it is useful to incorporate such a report format in the planning stages of the surveillance effort, recognizing that some unanticipated findings may cause a modification to the dissemination plan.

Depending on the size and makeup of the intended audience, it may be beneficial to use the media as a multiplier and plan to develop materials for them to use in writing articles. For instance, if certain management practices used by producers are found to influence disease occurrence, publications read by producers and veterinarians may offer the best means to communicate these findings. In this case, the communication would hopefully result in education of producers and veterinarians and ultimately lead to improved health status of the animals. In each of our NAHMS projects, we have attempted to assess from where the producer gets health-related information to continue to fine-tune the information dissemination effort. In some cases, the producer has looked most frequently to personnel in feed sales for animal health information, rather than to a book, magazine, or veterinary practitioner. In this case, it may well be that the best way to relay surveillance findings to some producers is via the feed stores and feed salespeople.

Timing of information dissemination is critical to its usefulness. Timing can also be critical in the order of dissemination. Many peer-reviewed publications will not accept a manuscript that does not present "new" information. If the findings from a project or surveillance system have been previously published in another external report, the journal may reject such material. In the NAHMS experience, it is best to get such items addressed by the editor of the journal on a case-by-case basis in advance. It may well be that rapid dissemination of groundbreaking animal health information in another format will preclude the possibility of publication in the peer-reviewed literature unless additional findings are reported. Advance planning can make this possible without sacrificing the timely dissemination of information for other audiences.

CONCLUSION

When designing a surveillance system, it is best to start with the end in mind. The information coming out of a surveillance system is generally expected to result in action and must reach the appropriate audience for action to occur. This chapter briefly describes the approaches used for NAHMS in the United States.

Danish Swine Salmonellosis Control Program: 1993 to 2001

J. Christensen

INTRODUCTION

In this chapter, the Danish Salmonellosis Control Program in swine (DSCP) is used as an example of a disease control process (Chapter 2). The description will start with detection of the *Salmonella* as a problem, and then some of the circumstances that influenced the decision to implement the DSCP will be presented. The DSCP as it was designed when first implemented (1995) and major changes to the program (1996–2001) will be described to illustrate that the program was a dynamic process in the years 1995 to 2001. Finally, the method applied to document the changes will be summarized.

Salmonella was first associated with disease in pigs in the nineteenth century by Salmon and Smith, but the infection in both animals and humans has probably been present for much longer. Since the nineteenth century, *Salmonella* spp. infections have been described for almost all vertebrae, frequently causing

Canadian Food Inspection Agency
Charlottetown, Prince Edward Island
Canada

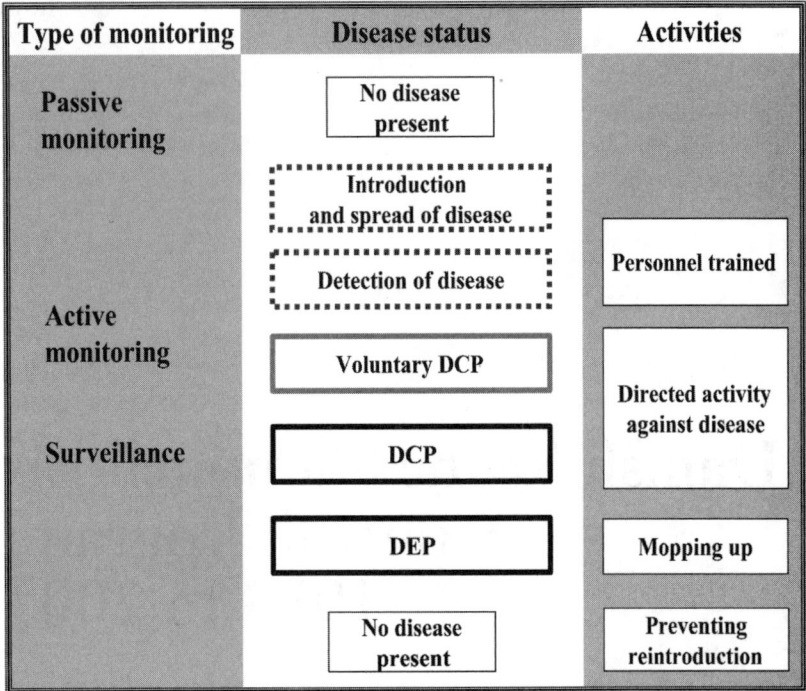

Type of monitoring	Disease status	Activities
Passive monitoring	No disease present	
	Introduction and spread of disease	
	Detection of disease	Personnel trained
Active monitoring	Voluntary DCP	Directed activity against disease
Surveillance	DCP	
	DEP	Mopping up
	No disease present	Preventing reintroduction

FIGURE 13.1   The disease control model: a visual model describing a disease control

disease. Therefore, we cannot say that domestic animal species have been free of infection and disease (Figure 13.1), but that *Salmonella* infections have not been regarded as a problem unless clinical disease reduced productivity (e.g., *Salmonella Choleraesuis*). Hence, Salmonellosis is an example of an endemic infectious disease in which a disease control process was initiated in swine after the problem was recognized.

PRIOR TO THE DANISH SALMONELLOSIS CONTROL PROGRAM (1993 AND 1994)

Salmonella spp. infection in Danish domestic swine has probably been present since swine were first commercially raised in the country.

DETECTION OF THE PROBLEM

In 1993, an epidemic of human Salmonellosis was detected in Denmark (Figure 13.2). The source of infection for this epidemic was traced back to a slaughter plant and to a few swineherds delivering slaughter pigs to that plant (Wegener

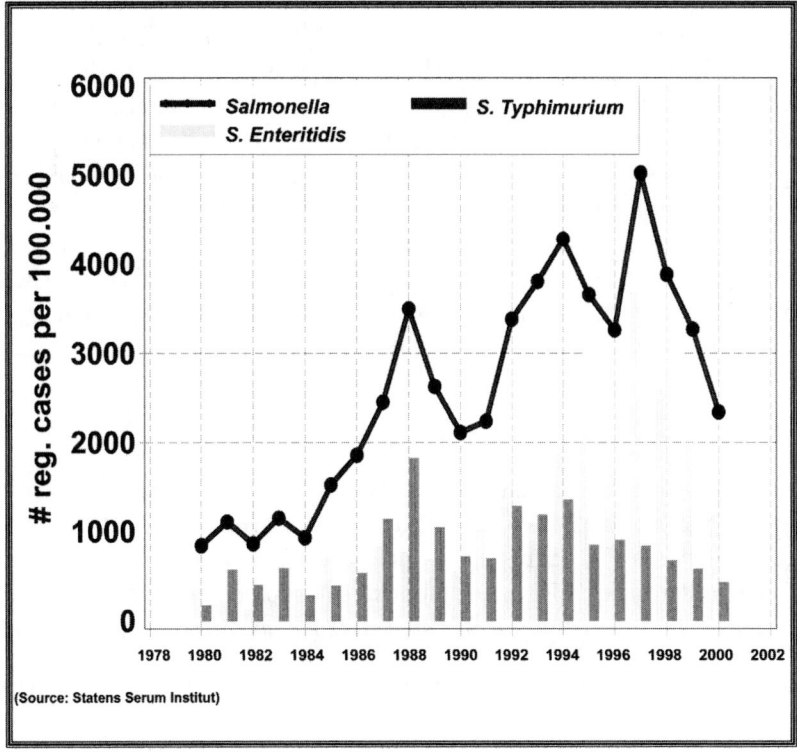

FIGURE 13.2   Registered cases of human Salmonellosis in Denmark 1980 to 2000.

and Baggesen, 1996). In 1993, *Salmonella infantis* infection in swine was considered a public human health risk.

CIRCUMSTANCES AND THEIR EFFECTS ON DECISIONS

The earlier outbreak in the late 1980s (Figure 13.2), attributed to chickens, had caused a decline in human consumption of poultry, and a Salmonellosis control program was implemented in broilers to restore consumer confidence in the Danish-produced poultry products. Media and politicians were very interested in the 1993 outbreak, and the public demanded that action be taken.

Although *Salmonella infantis* caused Salmonellosis in humans, the infection was largely subclinical in swine. Furthermore, Salmonellosis in swine was a well-known disease, but there were limited publications about prevention, control, and elimination of subclinical disease in swine. There was scientific uncertainty of the *Salmonella* culturing techniques as a large-scale diagnostic tool for subclinical disease. The prevalent occurrence of *Salmonella* infection in Danish swineherds was also unknown. The only monitoring of *Salmonella* in swineherds was the notification of clinical disease (i.e., passive collection of data for monitoring and surveillance systems [MOSSs]). Therefore, the situation may be described as one in which the politicians were faced with an unacceptable risk, scientific uncertainty, and public concerns (Commission of the European Communities, Anonymous 2000). Therefore, the precautionary principle was applied and the political decision was that all swine herds should be tested for *Salmonella*.

The immediate actions were to change from passive to active collection of data by use of bacteriologic surveys and monitoring of feed and pork, to develop diagnostic tests for large-scale monitoring, and to start a research program to gain knowledge of effective control measures for subclinical *Salmonella* spp. infection in swine.

Active Collection of Data for MOSS

A bacteriologic survey was initiated in 1993–1994, which included 1,363 swineherds. Ten cecal samples were collected from each herd, using slaughter animals. The findings from this survey indicated that *Salmonella* infection was present in all regions of Denmark, the apparent herd prevalence was 22%, and the most frequent serotype was *Salmonella typhimurium* (Baggesen et al. 1996).

Salmonella Reduction and Monitoring at the Feed Mill

Analogies to the Salmonellosis control program in broilers were drawn, and contaminated feed was considered a potential source of infection for swine. Therefore, heat treatment of feed for swine and monitoring of the feed process and of processed feed at all feed mills were initiated.

Monitoring of Pork

As part of the quality control at slaughterhouses, pork was examined for *Salmonella* contamination. The quality control was not designed to monitor *Salmonella* spp. prevalence, but the results were used as a national monitoring of the end product of the slaughtering process.

The following table depicts the design of this monitoring system:

Item	Description
Population	All export authorized slaughter plants in Denmark (from 1997 all slaughter plants).
Sample size	One sample per 200 slaughtered swine but at least one per month. At the national level, the sample size was about 2,200 samples per month.
Tissue samples	A variety of cuts and offal.
Diagnostic test	Bacterial culture for *Salmonella* spp.

Research Program (1994–1998)

The swine industry, specifically the Danish Bacon and Meat Council, the diagnostic laboratory (Danish Veterinary Institute [DVI]), the veterinary authority (Danish Veterinary and Food Administration [DVFA], and the Royal Veterinary and Agricultural University) launched a research program to reduce the scientific uncertainty about appropriate diagnostic tests and control or intervention measures. The research was principally funded by the Ministry and the Danish Bacon and Meat Council (DBMC), but all participating institutions funded specific portions of their own research.

Projects in the program investigated *Salmonella* contamination on infected farms, risk factors for subclinical *Salmonella* infection, vaccination, monitoring techniques, importance of healthy carriers, and intervention methods. The aim of the research was to incorporate new knowledge about MOSS into the DSCP as soon as it was available.

IMPLEMENTATION OF THE DSCP

PARTICIPANTS

Three foremost participants were responsible for the design and maintenance of the DSCP: the DVFA, the DBMC, and the DVI.

In Denmark, the infrastructure of the swine industry, veterinary authorities, and laboratory facilities work together, and no competition can be observed.

In the DVFA, one department has the responsibility for national disease control programs in livestock and another department is responsible for the quality control at slaughterhouses. The jurisdiction for these two departments is clearly defined. The legislative role rested with the DVFA, and as part of the Ministry, it represented the general public including the consumers.

The DBMC represented more than 95% of the total production of swine in Denmark. The organization is a cooperative entity that represents both swine producers and slaughterhouses. It collects specific fees from these groups, and the funding is spent on marketing, research, disease control, and support for farm consultations. There has been a long tradition for disease control and eradication initiated with strong support from the DBMC. For example, the specific-pathogen-free (SPF) system is part of the DBMC, and in the 1980s, the DBMC had been one of the main participants in the eradication of Aujeszky's Disease.

Even though competition existed among the individual slaughterhouse companies within the DBMC, their common interest was to restore consumer confidence in Danish-produced pork.

In 1993, Denmark had four laboratories doing diagnostic tests on materials from swineherds. The Danish Veterinary Institute for Virus Research (DVIV) was working with viral diseases, and the Danish Veterinary Laboratory (DVL) was responsible for diagnostic tests on production animals in general. DVIV and DVL were the national governmental veterinary diagnostic laboratories. Two other laboratories, a serologic laboratory mainly working with monitoring in the SPF-system (Roskilde) and a laboratory working with pathology, bacteriology, and parasitology (Kjellerup), were owned by the DBMC. Both laboratories participated in applied research, but they had limited diagnostic test development. All four laboratories had a close working relationship concerning routine diagnostic procedures. Both Kjellerup and DVL performed routine testing of samples from swineherds for *Salmonella* by culture, but DVL was the only laboratory responsible for serology as well as further typing of *Salmonella* isolates. Furthermore, a serologic test for detection of antibodies for *Salmonella* was under development at DVL. Therefore, DVL became a main participant in the DSCP.

POPULATION OF INTEREST

The foremost aim of the disease control process program is to reduce the risk to human health. Therefore, the principle of the disease control process was a stable-to-table approach. The DSCP in swine was intended to be a third link in the chain from stable to table (Figure 13.3), closing the gap between the farm and the slaughterhouse.

The slaughter pig population was viewed as the swine population with the closest link to exposure to humans through pork products. Furthermore, monitoring was seen as a quality control of the end product for the swine producers. It was assumed that if the prevalence of *Salmonella*-infected pigs were low enough when pigs arrived at the slaughter plant, infection in other age groups (e.g., sows) would not be a substantial risk to human health. Therefore, the livestock population of interest for the DSCP was the Danish slaughter pig herds.

MONITORING

Decisions about monitoring were based on epidemiologic and statistical calculations, as well as other circumstances. When the large-scale monitoring of the slaughter pig population in the DSCP was designed, the issues discussed were diagnostic assays, biologic specimens, the logistics of sampling, and the statistical considerations. For each of these issues, more options were considered; the main circumstances that influenced the decision are listed in Table 13.1.

Diagnostic Assays

Comparing the cost of testing using a Mix-ELISA system (Nielsen el al. 1995) with the cost of a culture for *Salmonella* was probably the most important fac-

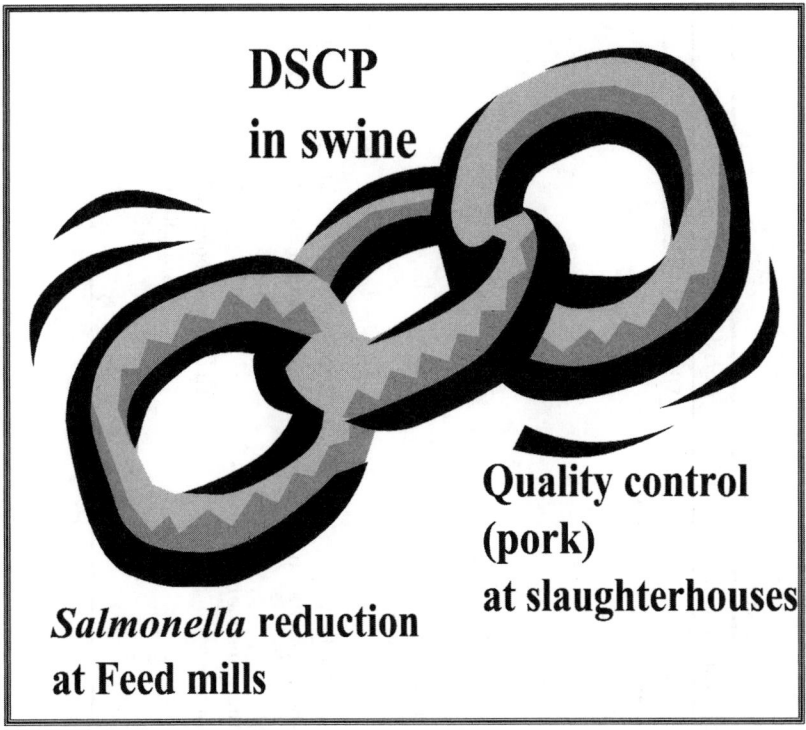

FIGURE 13.3   The complexity of the disease control process to reduce human exposure to *Salmonella* through Danish-produced pork that included three links. A part of this process was the Danish *Salmonella* Control Program.

tor in the decision. The cost of testing per sample using the ELISA was approximately US$2, and the cost of a culture including species identification for the same sample was at least US$20 (for additional typing, e.g., serotyping, the price would increase).

Furthermore, the ability to detect subclinical disease or healthy carriers of *Salmonella* was considered an important issue, and therefore, antibody detection was considered more sensitive at the herd level. Culturing was deemed to have low sensitivity of detection of *Salmonella* in subclinically infected animals or in intermittent fecal shedders of the bacteria.

Finally, the procedure to develop and operate the diagnostic assay (Mix-ELISA) including setting up diagnostic facilities for handling about one million samples annually was present at the DVL (Nielsen et al 1995). Thus, a decision was made to consider the mix-ELISA system as the diagnostic test in the monitoring of slaughter pig herds to detect antibodies against *Salmonella* O-antigens 1, 4, 5, 6, 7, and 12.

TABLE 13.1   The Design of Monitoring in the Danish Swine Salmonellosis Control Program

Issues considered	Choices	Circumstances with influence on decisions	Decision
Diagnostic method	a) Serological test (antibody detection) b) Culturing (*Salmonella* detection)	a) Cost of the test b) Ability to detect subclinical disease c) Expertise at laboratories	Mix enzyme-linked immunosorbent assay
Material for the diagnostic test	a) Blood or meat-juice (serological testing) b) Pen samples, feces, or cecal contents (culturing)	a) Diagnostic test b) Logistics of sampling c) Expertise at laboratories	Meat-juice
Sampling site	a) Farms b) Slaughter plants	a) Cost of sampling b) Infrastructure of the swine industry c) Expertise	Slaughter plants
Sampling sizes and frequency	a) Number of herds b) Number of pigs within herds c) Ongoing or repeated sampling	a) Political consideration b) Epidemiological and statistical calculations c) Practical and economic constraints	Ongoing sampling of all slaughter pig producing herds with an annual kill over 100 pigs
Data handling	a) DVFA b) DBMC c) Laboratories d) Slaughterhouses	a) Political consideration b) Expertise	The Danish Zoonosis Register owned by DVFA was an integrated Central Husbandry Register owned by the Ministry.

Abbreviations: DVFA, Danish Veterinary and Food Administration; DBMC, Danish Bacon and Meat Council.

Sampling Site

Sampling site was the next issue to be considered. The economic cost and the infrastructure of the swine industry were a major determinant for the selection choice of site. In 1995, there were about 20,000 swine herds and about 80 slaughter plants; therefore, sampling only 80 plants would be more cost-efficient than sampling 20,000 herds (note, as mentioned before, that the determination had been that all herds should be included) if the appropriate diagnostic test and sampling technique could be found.

Expertise in the collection of blood from swineherds would exist only with veterinary practitioners, but at slaughterhouses, technicians could directly collect blood. Therefore, sampling at the slaughter plants would also reduce the cost of manpower as labor costs for technicians were cheaper than for veterinarians.

Biologic Specimens for the Diagnostic Test

The needed sample for the Mix-ELISA is serum usually extracted from blood samples. There was however, a problem with blood samples taken at the slaughter line. The blood samples can be obtained at exsanguination or as heart samples at the veterinary inspection station, but each option presented problems. At the exsanguination, the pigs were not readily identifiable because the slap-tatoo is invisible before scalding. Therefore, the pigs could not be traced back to the herd of origin, which was the purpose of the monitoring. At the veterinary inspection station, the pigs could be traced back to the herd, but the blood obtained from the heart had poor quality for serum extraction and the ELISA test. Furthermore, the blood tended to homogenize or rapidly deteriorate because it was taken after scalding.

When the mix-ELISA was adapted to serum extracted from meat (Nielsen et al. 1998), the possibility of using meat samples presents a possible solution to the problem of sampling serum at slaughter plants. Meat samples could be collected at the scale, where the identification of each pig was read and entered into the administrative systems of the slaughterhouse for payment of the swine producer.

Meat samples were easy to sample, and the cost of sampling by technicians could be kept low compared with blood sampling by veterinarians.

Sample Size

The sample size and sampling frequency were determined by the political decision that all swine herds should be tested for *Salmonella*, epidemiologic and statistical factors, and practical and economic constraints.

The epidemiologic and statistical sample size considerations were published in 1997. A stratified random sampling scheme, in which herds were stratified by expected annual slaughter, was applied (Table 13.2).

TABLE 13.2   The Danish Swine Salmonellosis Control Program: Sampling
Scheme and Intervention Thresholds for the Serologic Monitoring of *Salmonella enterica* Infections in Danish Slaughter Pig Herds (1995 to 2001)

Estimated number of finishers per year	Sample size of the expected annual kill (%)	Within-herd intervention prevalence (%)		Prevalence (%) detection limit*
		Level 2	Level 3	
1–100	0	—	—	—
101–200	11.1†	> 50	> 50	48.7
201–500	9.9	25–50	> 50	10.0
501–1,000	7.2	23–50	> 50	6.7
1,001–2,000	4.3	20–50	> 50	5.6
2,001–3,000	3.3	20–50	> 50	4.4
3,001–5,000	3.3	17–50	> 50	2.8
> 5,001	3.5	10–33	> 33	1.3

* Prevalence at which the confidence of detecting one positive pig per year is at least 95%.

† Since June 1997, increased to 25%.

Note. From Christensen et al. 1999.

Practical and economic constraints limited the sampling to herds with an expected slaughter of over 100 pigs per year. The small herds (less than 100 slaughtered annually) would contribute very little to the total amount of pork produced in Denmark, and therefore, their contribution to the human health risk was deemed negligible.

INTERVENTION THRESHOLDS

Two intervention thresholds for infected herds were defined by a herd-level diagnostic test (Christensen and Gardner 2000). The herd test was applied each month to classify herds into three levels: low and acceptable seroprevalence, moderate seroprevalence, and high and unsatisfactory seroprevalence (Christensen et al. 1999). The herd-level diagnostic test can be summarized as shown in Box 13.1.

INTERVENTIONS

In 1995, the interventions were predefined at slaughter (second intervention threshold) and on farms (first intervention threshold).

Slaughter

Slaughter of the animals is required for level-3 herds, and it has to be supervised by the DVFA. The intervention includes special hygiene precaution, which is demanded for all pigs originating from level-3 herds. Furthermore, an additional

> ## Box 13.1
>
> *Within-herd sample:* All test results from the herd within the last 3 months. Sample size depended on herd size (Table 13.2; Mousing et al. 1997; Christensen et al. 1999).
>
> *Diagnostic test:* Mix-enzyme-linked immunosorbent assay (Nielsen et al. 1998).
>
> *Individual test cutoff:* OD% = 40 equal to OD value = 30 (Christensen et al. 1999).
>
> *Herd level cutoff for level 2:*
> * First intervention threshold: 10% to 50% positive samples (Table 13.2).
>
> *Herd level cutoff for level 3:*
> * Second intervention threshold: 33% to 50% positive samples (Table 13.2).

quality control prescribed that carcasses from batches of level-3 herds were bacteriologically tested for *Salmonella* to assess the level of cross contamination. If the bacteriologic results were unacceptable (i.e., above 2.5% of the samples were *Salmonella* positive), the whole batch was heat treated or salted.

On Farm

The DBMC had additional requirements for their swine producers in both levels 2 and 3. The requirement intervention was that the producer must call a practicing veterinarian and a local swine specialist to determine an appropriate intervention strategy to reduce the seroprevalence. In addition, a 3-month follow-up visit is demanded by the DBMC.

The first intervention threshold (level 2) and the interventions urged by the DBMC may be considered a voluntary program instituted by a group of producers and slaughterhouses. However, the DBMC was almost a monopoly organization, with more than 95% of the total production and herds, so the individual swine producers may not have considered it a voluntary program.

Data Handling

The infrastructure of existing national databases and political considerations influence the decisions about the logistics of data handling in the DSCP.

In 1992, the Ministry had established the General Agricultural Register (GLR) and the Central Husbandry Register (CHR). The GLR maintains data related to the owner and location on all farm premises in Denmark, whereas the CHR maintains data related to animal production and herd size and so forth.

Slaughterhouses that were members of the DBMC had an administrative system to assist payment of producers and to report veterinary inspection data to the producers.

For political reasons, the Zoonosis Register (ZOOR) is government owned to secure public access to all data. ZOOR was established as a part of CHR, and thereby, ZOOR was owned by the DVFA, which represented the Ministry.

In summary, ZOOR linked data from CHR, the slaughterhouses, laboratories, and the DVFA to assist calculating sample size for the individual herd, sampling at the slaughter plants, handling of results and findings data, and assigning *Salmonella* herd level and its potential restrictions.

Voluntary Programs

As previously mentioned, the on-farm intervention measures may be considered a voluntary control program. The disease control programs implemented by the Breeders Association under the DBMC (DanAvl) and Pig Improvement Company (PIC) are both examples of such volunteer optional programs.

The voluntary program instituted by the breeding organizations in Denmark was an addition to the meat-juice screening and is not considered an alternative to the screening. The monitoring for this voluntary program is similar to the monitoring of slaughter swineherds, except blood samples from the herds were used in the herd-level test and a weighted average (*Salmonella* index) was introduced as described in Box 13.2.

The intervention was restrictive on sale and movement of breeding stock, and the DBMC recommends consulting visits to advise on a strategy to reduce the *Salmonella* seroprevalence.

Box 13.2

Within-herd sample: 10 blood samples from gilts 4-7 months of age per month.

Diagnostic test: Mix-enzyme-linked immunosorbent assay (Nielsen et al. 1996).

Herd-level test result:
- *Salmonella* index: A weighted average of OD% of all test results from the herd within the last 3 months. The monthly average OD values were weighted 6:3:1.

Herd level cutoff:
- Intervention threshold: *Salmonella* index > 15.

CHANGES TO THE DSCP (1996–2001)

The DSCP has never been a static program because minor changes and adjustments have been made continuously throughout the years. For example, in 1997, the sample size for the small herds increased from 11% to 25% (Table 13.2) because of the fact that these herds had irregular shipments of swine to slaughter, and they often would be placed in level 3 on the basis of one positive sample. Another example from the voluntary program was that the breeding companies would notify their members if the *Salmonella* index was greater than five.

It is beyond the scope of this chapter to document all changes in the DSCP over the years; therefore, only some of the important changes in monitoring (Figure 13.4) and intervention measures (Figure 13.5) will be addressed.

Follow-up Bacteriologic Testing

In 1996, bacteriologic follow-up testing in herds that were in both levels 2 or 3 was implemented and was mandatory. The follow-up was an improvement of the monitoring at the national level and an intervention at the herd level.

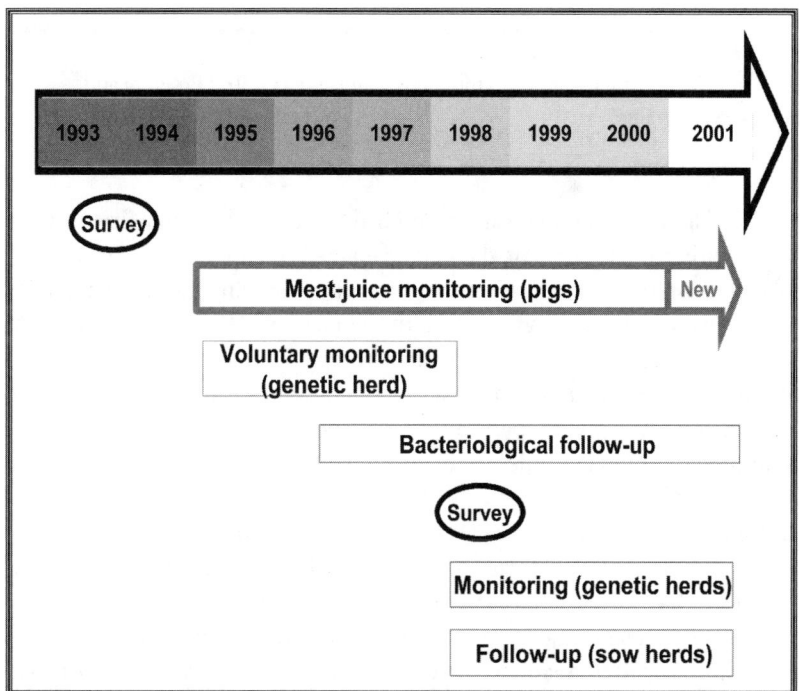

FIGURE 13.4   Monitoring in the Danish *Salmonella* Control Program and related surveys.

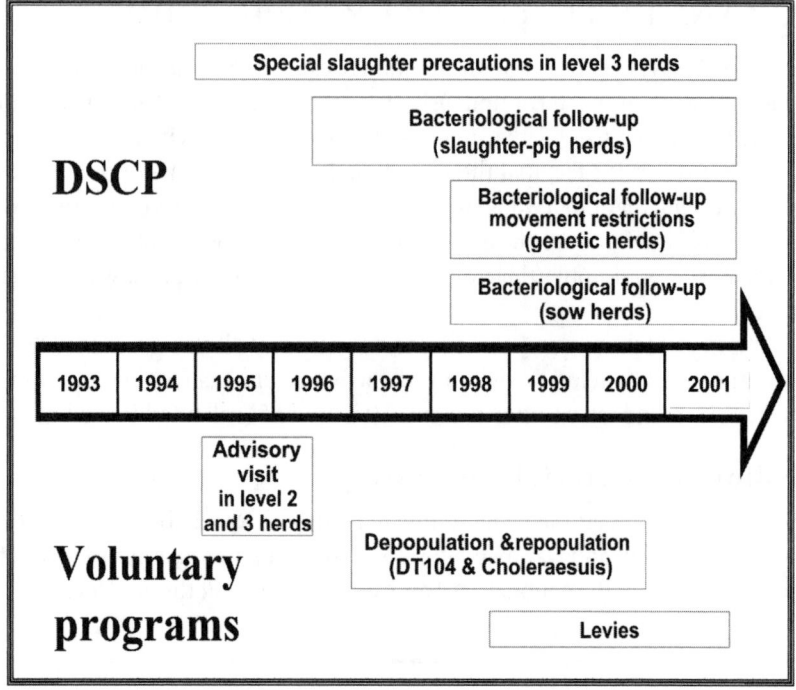

FIGURE 13.5   Interventions in the Danish *Salmonella* Control Program and voluntary programs.

The follow-up examination was applied to herds when they first were assigned either level 2 or 3 or the herd remained in either level 2 or 3 after 3 months from their classification. A swine producer being informed about the follow-up program was referred to as "the injunction." The aim of the follow-up in the infected herds was to identify the serotype(s) present and identify the infected portion of the production system units. Within 35 days of the injunction, at least five pooled pen samples should be collected for culture, and representative blood samples were recommended but optional.

The producer is responsible for the cost of the collection of the specimens and shipment of samples. The DVFA is responsible for the cost of the laboratory's expenses (culturing, serotyping, and ELISA testing). The DVFA could fine herds that did not comply with the follow-up program.

The individual swine producer would consider the follow-up sampling as an extra expense and thus, an incentive to improve control of Salmonellosis. The local veterinarian would use the follow-up as a tool in the consultant service to the herd owner because it would give insight into the serotypes present in the herd and help locate the problem in specific production units. Therefore, at the herd level, the follow-up could be viewed as an intervention measure and a motivation of the entire program.

At the national level, the follow-up program was an intensified monitoring of Salmonellosis because it provided information about the diversity of serotypes in the Danish swine population.

The decision to implement the follow-up program was influenced by scientific, practical, and legal issues. From the scientific point, the follow-up program would allow us to monitor the diversity of serotypes to ensure that the mix-ELISA can detect the predominant serotypes (with their O-antigens). Practically, swine producers need a stronger motivation to control Salmonellosis in their infected herds. The previous consequences of a moderate or high seroprevalence in the herd (level 2 or level 3) were that the DBMC demanded consultancy visits, but it was the choice of the producer to follow the advice. Therefore, it was decided that legislation should support the activities in the infected herds. It was deemed legally impossible to fine and sue producers for not following advice but possible to sue them for not having samples taken. Therefore, the follow-up program was a practical solution to improve motivation and monitoring in the DSCP.

EXPANSION OF THE DSCP

The next major changes to DSCP were implemented in 1998. These changes followed an internal scrutiny of the DSCP as a result of an increased number of human cases attributed to *Salmonella enteritidis* in table eggs in 1997 (Figure 13.2) and detection of multi-drug resistant *Salmonella typhimurium* DT104 in the swine population. Increased political and media attention to Salmonellosis in the Danish livestock production, specifically broilers, table eggs, and swine, had worked to speed up the process to implement the changes.

The aim of the changes was to extend the population of interest to the whole swine population and to improve the monitoring of multi-drug resistant *Salmonella typhimurium* DT104. Therefore, the new activities were aimed at breeding and stock herds (referred to as genetic herds), specialized sow herds, and increased bacteriologic follow-up in moderate- or high-seroprevalence herds.

Breeding and Genetic Herds
The voluntary program with monitoring and monthly collection of blood samples was modified and included in the DSCP (Figure 13.4) as shown in Box 13.3.

Sow Herds
Specialized sow herds, defined as herds of weaned piglets (7 to 30 kg) and producing less than 100 slaughter pigs per year, had not been monitored in the

---

Box 13.3

Within-herd sample: Monthly collection of 10 blood samples from gilts 4–7 months of age per each month.

Diagnostic test: Mix-enzyme-linked immunosorbent assay (Nielsen et al. 1996).

Herd-level test result:
- *Salmonella* index: A weighted average of OD% of all test results from the herd within the last 3 months. The monthly average OD values were weighted 6:3:1.

Herd level cutoffs:
- First intervention threshold: *Salmonella* index > 5.
- Second intervention threshold: *Salmonella* index > 15.

Interventions:
- First intervention threshold: mandatory bacteriological follow-up— within 35 days, at least five pooled pen samples should be collected for culture. Blood samples were recommended but optional.
- Second intervention threshold: restriction on sale and movement of breeding stock.

DSCP prior to 1998. The main justification was that these herds had not been defined as the population of interest. In addition, monitoring these herds presented a scientific and an economic problem. Scientifically, a serologic diagnostic test suited for the age groups in these herds was not available. The mix-ELISA was not deemed accurate enough for monitoring sows because this test had proven difficult in determining an individual diagnostic test cutoff for sows, and the 7- to 30-kg piglets would not have developed antibodies to the infection. Therefore, the far more expensive process of monitoring by repeated herd examination by culture seemed to be the only method available.

The acceptable option that maintains reasonable cost of monitoring sow herds is to target the monitoring of high-risk herds. High-risk herds are those with a history of trade contact with infected slaughter pig herds. Therefore, the monitoring implemented in the sow herds was a bacteriologic follow-up testing in herds delivering pigs (7 to 30 kg) to slaughter-pig producing herds in both levels 2 and 3 (Figure 13.4). The scheme is depicted in Box 13.4.

Note that in the sow herds, no general surveillance for *Salmonella* in general was introduced because there were no intervention threshold or predefined in-

---

Box 13.4

Selection of sow herds: All herds that shipped pigs (7 to 30 kg) to slaughter-pig producing herds in levels 2 or 3.

Method of selection: Mandatory reporting of herd of origin of all pigs (7 to 30 kg) 6 months before the assignment of levels 2 or 3.

Sample size:
- Mandatory bacteriological follow-up: within 35 days, at least five pooled pen samples should be collected for culture.

---

terventions. However, there was a specific surveillance system for multi-drug resistant *Salmonella typhimurium* DT104.

Multi-drug Resistant *Salmonella Typhimurium* DT104

Improved surveillance for multi-drug resistant *Salmonella typhimurium* DT104 was achieved by the intensified follow-up in herds with moderate or high seroprevalence or their contact herds. The follow-up served as a herd-level diagnostic test for multi-drug resistant *Salmonella typhimurium* DT104 (see Box 13.5).

Special Survey in 1998

The appropriate control strategy for multi-drug resistant *Salmonella typhimurium* DT104 in swineherds was debated because of the uncertainty of its prevalence. Therefore, a survey with bacteriologic testing was carried out in 1998. The survey comprised a random sample of slaughter pig producing herds ($N = 1,962$); a random sample of farrow-to-grower (sow) herds ($N = 305$); and all breeding and genetic herds ($N = 366$). The previous bacteriologic study on *Salmonella* occurrence was in 1993 through 1994 (Baggesen et al. 1996) and served as a model for the study design. The conclusion of the survey was that the prevalence of multi-drug resistant *Salmonella typhimurium* DT104 was lower in the examined slaughter swineherds than in the other herds. (Christensen et al. 2002; Figure 13.4).

Voluntary Programs

The DBMC implemented additional intervention measures in their member herds. In general, a stronger economic incentive to reduce the *Salmonella* occurrence in level-3 herds was introduced by the slaughterhouse companies. These companies demanded a special levy on every pig slaughtered from herds

---

BOX 13.5

Selection of herds:
1   Breeding and genetic herds with *Salmonella* index greater than 5;
2   Slaughter-pig herds in level 2 or level 3;
3   Sow herds that sold pigs to slaughter pig herds in level 2 or level 3.

Within-herd sample: At least five pooled pen samples (10 pools were recommended)

Diagnostic test: Culture and serotyping of isolates.

Herd level cutoff:
• Intervention threshold: One isolate of multi-drug resistant *Salmonella typhimurium* DT104.

Interventions:
• Trade and movement restrictions
• Special hygiene precautions at slaughter

Further actions: Identification of contact herds and examination of their Salmonellosis status by 40–50 pooled pen samples.

---

in level 3. The levy depended on how long the herd had high seroprevalence. Since 1998, the levies have been gradually increased.

An eradication strategy for multi-drug resistant *Salmonella typhimurium* DT104 and *Salmonella Choleraesuis* was pursued. Starting in 1997, the herds that had been diagnosed with multi-drug resistant *Salmonella typhimurium* DT104 were enrolled in an eradication program. The infected herd was depopulated and repopulated and subsequently examined for multi-drug resistant *Salmonella typhimurium* DT104 in an elaborate testing scheme. Similarly, three herds diagnosed with *Salmonella Choleraesuis* were depopulated and repopulated following the same protocol.

These eradication programs were an example of a modified precautionary principle applied by the swine industry, and they were adopted until additional knowledge of occurrence could be obtained.

REVISION OF THE CONTROL STRATEGY

The continued progress in a control program with some success depends on revision of the short- and long-term goals. The overall goal of the Salmonellosis control process was revised for the first time in 1999.

New Control Strategy for Salmonellosis (1999–2001)

In 1999, an agreement between the Ministry and the DBMC revised the goals of the Salmonellosis control process. The short-term target was to have a prevalence of *Salmonella* in pork was under 1% by the end of 1999 and 0.5% by the end of 2001. The long-term goal was that the occurrence in pork should be as close to zero as practically and scientifically possible. Ongoing adjustments of the entire Salmonellosis control process from stable to table were expected.

New Control Strategy for DT104 (2000)

In a report related to multi-drug resistant *Salmonella typhimurium* DT104, the DVFA, DVL, and DBMC compiled the new science-based knowledge about occurrence, intervention, and control measures possible in herds and during the slaughter process. The recommendation in the report was to end the eradication strategy and adopt a control strategy. In addition, recommendations were made to first improve the herd-level diagnostic test in the serologic monitoring by adjusting the samples sizes and cutoffs to adapt to a lower seroprevalence in 2000 than in 1995. The objective of these changes was to obtain an earlier detection of herds infected with multi-drug resistant *Salmonella typhimurium* DT104$. Second, recommendations were made to implement zoonosis restrictions in herds diagnosed with multi-drug resistant *Salmonella typhimurium* DT104. The restrictions included measures related to trade and movement of animals and products thereof, manure management, and implementation of measures to reduce *Salmonella* occurrence.

The above changes were fully implemented by the end of 2000.

MONITORING FRESH PORK (2001)

Salmonella prevalence in pork became the success parameter in 1999, but the existing monitoring was deemed inadequate to measure changes in prevalence as low as 0.5% to 1%. Therefore, a new monitoring method for pork was designed and tested. The scheme for this monitoring method is outlined in Box 13.6.

From autumn 1999 to spring 2000, the new and existing monitoring methods were conducted in parallel in nine slaughter plants to document the accuracy of the new method as compared with the old one. The new monitoring method was more sensitive than the old method; therefore, a correction factor of 1.9 was calculated to allow comparison of the prevalence in pork before and after implementation of the new monitoring method.

The new monitoring of pork was fully implemented from January 2001 (Figure 13.4).

Box 13.6

Material: Swabs of chilled carcasses.

Sample size: Five carcasses per day per export authorized slaughter plant and five carcasses per 200 pigs in other slaughter plants (at least five carcasses per month).

Diagnostic test: Culture of pools of five swabs.

Intervention threshold:
- Export authorized slaughter plants: two positive tests within 11 days.
- Other slaughter plants: one positive test

Intervention: Scrutiny of the slaughter process to identify hygiene failure breakdown.

MEAT-JUICE SCREENING (2001)

The meat-juice screening had remained largely unchanged from 1995 to 2000, when it was decided to review the sampling scheme, individual- and herd-level cutoff, and intervention thresholds. The motivation for the review was that the *Salmonella* prevalence had declined to about 3% in 1998 to 2000 (Figure 13.6), and no further decline was expected if strict criteria for classifying problem herds were not introduced. The declining prevalence also made it more difficult to detect *Salmonella* in the follow-up examination, and therefore, it was desired to have the follow-up examination earlier in the infection stage in the herds. Finally, similar changes were recommended in the *Salmonella typhimurium* DT104 report.

The new classification system was implemented in August 2001, as outlined in Box 13.7.

DOCUMENTATION OF CHANGES

The changes in the DSCP were documented in six internal reports (in Danish). In the reports, the status of disease occurrence, summary of knowledge acquired since the last evaluation, and changes in circumstances was followed by an evaluation of the progress, success parameters, and fulfillment of short and long-term goals. The reports then recommended a revision of the following items: control strategy and short and long-term goals, monitoring, interven-

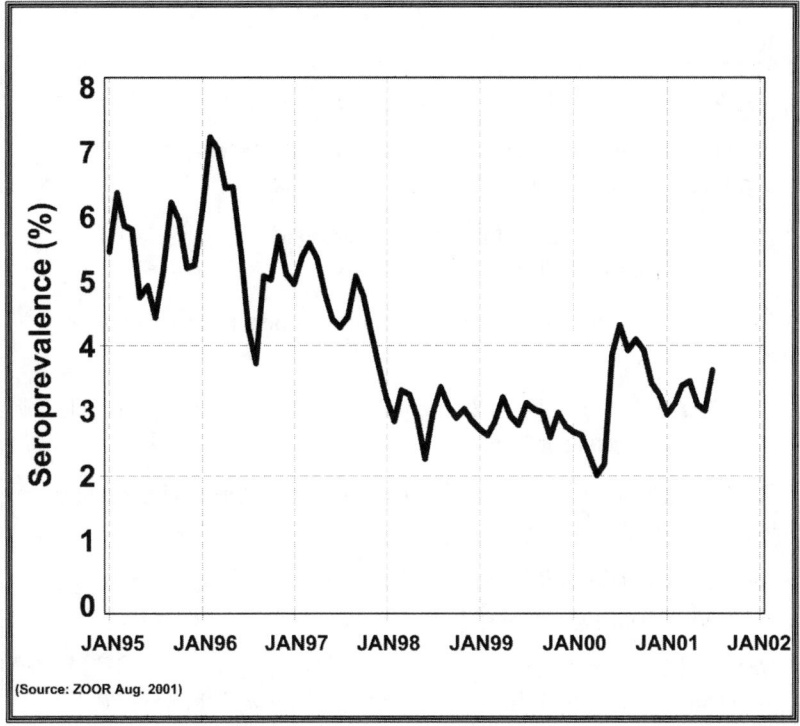

FIGURE 13.6   Seroprevalence in the meat-juice screening of the Danish *Salmonella* Control Program.

tion thresholds, and intervention measures. Finally, the expected costs were calculated and suggestions for financing were made.

In general, the changes were supported by scientifically based knowledge gained from research carried out by the participants and other institutions. Most changes were implemented as soon as internal reports from the research projects provided adequate recommendation. For example, more independent studies demonstrated that important risk factors for *Salmonella* were related to feed and feeding systems. Later, some of the results of projects were published at conferences or in peer-reviewed journals.

DEFINITIONS APPLIED IN THE DSCP

- **Breeding and multiplying herds:** members of DanAvl or PIC. Same as genetic herds.

Box 13.7

Population of interest: Herds with an expected slaughter over 200 swine.

Within-herd sample size: The annual sample size is 60, 75, or 100 depending on herd size (Alban et al. 2001).

Within-herd sample: All test results from the herd within the last 3 months (Alban et al. 2001).

Diagnostic test: Mix-enzyme-linked immunosorbent assay (Nielsen et al. 1998).

Individual test cutoff: OD% = 20 is equal to OD value = 10 (Alban et al. 2001; Christensen et al. 1999).

Serologic Salmonella index: Weighted average (0.2;0.2;0.6) of seroprevalence over the last 3 months.

Herd level cutoff for level 2:
• First intervention threshold: serologic *Salmonella* index = 40.

Herd level cutoff for level 3:
• Second intervention threshold: serologic *Salmonella* index = 70.

• **Follow-up program:** An integrated (from August 1996) part of the *Salmonella* Control Program concerned with the follow-up in subclinically infected herds (moderate or high seroprevalence based on meat-juice screening), and for members of the DBMC, it also included interventions in the individual herds.
• **Follow-up:** Bacteriologic examination of pooled pen samples.
• **Genetic herds:** Members of DanAvl or PIC. Same as breeding and multiplying herds.
• **Injunction:** The event where herd owners are informed that their herd has been categorized into level 2 or 3, that they have to comply with the follow-up program, and about penalties if they do not comply with the program.
• **Level:** *Salmonella* level of a herd based on the 3-month moving average seroprevalence measured by examination (mix-ELISA) of meat-juice samples taken from pigs at slaughter. This level is assigned every month.
• **Meat-juice screening:** The ongoing screening of all Danish slaughter-pig herds with an expected kill above 100 pigs per year for the occurrence of *Salmonella* using meat-juice samples at slaughter.

- **OD%:** Calibrated optical densities obtained through regression analyses on ODs of positive- and negative-reference sera and expressed as OD%.
- **OD value:** Optical density values coded as: OD% − 10 and censored at 1. That is, all samples with an OD% below 12 had an OD value of 1, and samples with an OD% of 12 or above had an OD value of OD% − 10. Zero was the code for missing test results.
- **Serologic** *Salmonella* index: Weighted average OD% over 3 months, applied in the monitoring of breeding and multiplying herds.
- **Seroprevalence:** Refers to prevalence measured by examination (mix-ELISA) of serum from meat-juice or blood samples.
- **Sow herds:** Herds selling pigs (7 to 30 kg) to slaughter-pig-producing herds.
- **Slaughter-pig herds:** Herds selling pigs for slaughter.

BIBLIOGRAPHY

Alban L., Stege H., Dahl J. 2001. The new classification system for slaughter-pig herds in the Danish *Salmonella* surveillance-and-control program. Prev Vet Med 53:133–146.

Anonymous. 2000. Commission of the European Communities, 2000. Communication from the Commission on the precautionary principle. Brussels 02.02.2000 COM(2000).

Baggesen D.L., Wegener H.C., Bager F., Stege H., Christensen J. 1996. Herd prevalence of *Salmonella enterica* infections in Danish slaughter pigs determined by microbiological testing. Prev Vet Med 26:201–213.

Christensen, J. 2001. Epidemiological concepts regarding disease monitoring and surveillance. Acta Vet Scand 94:11–16.

Christensen J., Gardner I.A. 2000. Herd-level interpretation of test results for epidemiologic studies of animal diseases. Prev Vet Med 45:83–106.

Christensen J., Baggesen D.L., Nielsen B., Stryhn H. 2002. Herd prevalence of *Salmonella* spp. in Danish pig herds after implementation of the Danish *Salmonella* Control Program with reference to a pre-implementation study. Vet Microbiol 88:175–188.

Christensen J., Baggesen D.L., Soerensen V., Svensmark B. 1999. *Salmonella* level of Danish swine herds based on serological examination of meat-juice samples and *Salmonella* occurrence measured by bacteriological follow-up. Prev Vet Med 40:277–292.

Nielsen B., Baggesen D.L., Bager F., Haugegaard J., Lind P. 1995. The serological response to *Salmonella* serovars *Typhimurium* and *Infantis* in experimentally infected pigs. The time course followed with an indirect anti-LPS ELISA and bacteriological examinations. Vet Microbiol 47:205–218.

Nielsen B., Ekeroth L., Bager F., Lind P. 1998. Use of muscle fluid as a source of antibodies for serologic detection of *Salmonella* infection in slaughter pig herds. J Vet Diag Invest 10:158–163.

Wegener H.C., Baggesen D.L. 1996. Investigation of an outbreak of human salmonellosis cause by *Salmonella enterica* serovar *infantis* by use of pulsed field gel electrophoresis. Int J Food Microbiol 32:125–131

Index

Page references given in *italics* refer to tables